COPING WITH
PROSTATE CANCER

Coping With

Prostate Cancer

Robert H. Phillips, Ph.D.

Avery Publishing Group
Garden City Park, New York

The medical information and procedures described in this book are not intended as a substitute for consulting your physician. All matters regarding your physical health should be supervised by a medical professional.

Cover Design: Ann Vestal
In-House Editor: Joanne Abrams
Original Illustrations: Nuno Faìsca
Typesetter: Bonnie Freid
Printer: Paragon Press, Honesdale, PA

Library of Congress Cataloging-in-Publication Data

Phillips, Robert H., 1948–
    Coping with prostate cancer : a guide to living with prostate cancer for you and your family / Robert H. Phillips.
      p. cm.
    Includes bibliographical references.
    ISBN 0-89529-564-4
    1. Prostate—Cancer. I. Title.
RC280.P7P48 1994
362.1'9699463—dc20
                                   93-43373
                                   CIP

Printed in the United States of America

10 9 8 7 6 5 4 3 2

CONTENTS

This book is lovingly dedicated to my family—
my wife, Sharon, and my three sons, Michael, Larry, and Steven;
my parents and sister; and all my other relatives and in-laws—
and to my friends.

This book is also affectionately dedicated to my four beloved grandparents,
now all gone, but never to be forgotten:
to the Kurzrocks—Bertha and Mickey—
and to the Phillipses—Gertrude and Charles—
my eternal gratitude for the love, guidance, and support
that was always unhesitatingly there for me.
I miss you!

ACKNOWLEDGMENTS

Appreciative words of thanks must be accorded to some very special people who provided assistance in the preparation of this book. Thanks to Lawrence Fish, M.D., for his helpful suggestions, his knowledgeable review of the manuscript, and his continuing belief in the project. Thanks to Ann Dominger, Melissa Sheinwold, and Carmela Vecchio for the hours spent transcribing, revising, and typing the manuscript. And thanks to Joanne Abrams, my editor at Avery Publishing Group, for her diligent work and valuable comments.

PREFACE

The diagnosis of prostate cancer can have a major impact on you and your family. No kidding! Many people shudder when they just hear the word "cancer." Fortunately, thanks to advances in modern medicine, many types of cancer can now be controlled and controlled well, allowing individuals to lead long, productive, happy lives. Of course, this doesn't mean that having prostate cancer is any less frightening. There are many people who, despite knowing the increased survival and cure rates, still worry that they will be among the unfortunate statistics.

Certainly, there are many misconceptions, fears, concerns, and myths about cancer and its treatment. You probably have many questions about prostate cancer. Some of them can be answered by physicians or other professionals. Others can be answered by the relatively few books or articles on the subject. However, many questions cannot be answered. Why? Scientists just don't know all the answers. This can be upsetting. Also upsetting is the feeling you may experience because you're dealing with the "C" word. And knowing that you have a chronic medical problem can be depressing.

In living with prostate cancer, you'll find yourself facing a number of important decisions. Initially, one of the most essential decisions you'll be making concerns how you can best become a partner in the treatment program that's going to help you, and how you can take control over the rest of your life, rather than letting life control you.

Heavy stuff? You bet it is! But that's why this book was written. Chock-full of information, suggestions, and strategies, this book will help you, your family, and your friends learn how to cope with prostate cancer.

The first two parts of the book present basic information about prostate cancer: what it is, what the symptoms are, what treatment techniques are available, and so on. The other parts of the book deal with important aspects of living with prostate cancer, including coping with emotions, making lifestyle changes, and living with others. We will

Coping With Prostate Cancer

explore each aspect in detail, and will examine many suggestions and strategies, as well as illustrative examples. In fact, a lot of the information you'll be reading can (and does!) apply to any chronic medical condition. In this book, however, the main focus is on your life with prostate cancer.

As you learn to cope with prostate cancer, it's important to realize that you're not alone; others are experiencing a lot of the same things that you're going through. This can be reassuring. But you should also remember that each person with prostate cancer experiences symptoms, as well as treatments, differently. Similarly, the psychological consequences of having prostate cancer vary from person to person. Your own life with prostate cancer—the way it affects you and the way you experience it—will not be exactly the same as anyone else's. You are a unique person. Therefore it will be up to *you* to use the suggestions and strategies presented in this book to help yourself cope as well as you possibly can. The goal of this book is to help you to become an active person, rather than a passive patient.

The American Cancer Society categorizes cancer as a chronic illness, not a terminal illness. A chronic illness is defined as one that is long lasting. It is a disorder that may create disability or handicap, requiring rehabilitation and ongoing supervision. Even when individuals are in remission, they may still need ongoing care. But because cancer is categorized this way, it suggests that dying is not the issue. The issue is learning how to live with the disease.

Until such time as there is no longer a condition called prostate cancer, you'll have to live with it. I hope this book will help both you and your family do just that, and do it comfortably. Remember: You can *always* improve the quality of your life.

Robert H. Phillips, Ph.D.
Center for Coping
Long Island, NY

PART I

PROSTATE CANCER— AN OVERVIEW

Chapter 1

THE PROSTATE—
IN A NUTSHELL

Jack, a fifty-eight-year-old insurance broker, had not been feeling well. He had been having trouble urinating for a couple of years, and was now experiencing pains that he had never felt before.

Finally, Jack went to his physician. His doctor gave him a complete physical examination, including blood and urine tests, and asked him very specific questions about his urination problems. Then the doctor's experienced fingers carefully probed Jack's pelvic area and gave him a digital rectal examination. Not liking what he felt, he performed a biopsy of Jack's prostate gland.

A few days later, the doctor sat down at his desk and prepared to discuss his findings with Jack. Jack nervously approached the chair by the doctor's desk and sat down, with his wife of twenty years at his side. The doctor looked at him and wasted no time in telling him, "Jack, you have prostate cancer." Jack's immediate reaction was very similar to the initial response of many individuals diagnosed with this condition. Trembling, he looked at the doctor and exclaimed, "Cancer???"

So what exactly is prostate cancer? In order to really understand prostate cancer, it's best to begin by talking about the prostate gland. The prostate is an accessory sex gland of the male reproductive system. This means that its function is to assist in the male reproductive process. Let's discuss the location, shape, size, structure, and function of this gland.

THE LOCATION AND SHAPE OF THE PROSTATE GLAND

The word *prostate* is a derivation of two Greek words. One is the preposition meaning "before," and the other is a verb that means "to stand." The prostate was so named because it "stands" before the bladder. The small conical gland is located right outside and below the outlet of the bladder, next to the wall of the rectum. You might picture the prostate as a tiny apple that's had its core removed. Passing through the prostate, much as the core would be found in the center of an apple, is the urethra—the tube that carries urine from the bladder out of the body through the penis. Also passing through the prostate is the ejaculatory duct, a narrow tube that is less than one inch long. This duct goes through the prostate and opens into the urethra. Ducts coming from the prostate itself also open into the urethra next to the ejaculatory duct openings. (See Figure 1.1.)

The prostate is located very close to large blood vessels and nerves that are important for the functioning of the penis. This location isn't a problem with a healthy prostate gland. But, as you'll read shortly, it may cause concern for people with prostate cancer. Why? If surgery is selected as a treatment, these blood vessels may be endangered, and any damage to the blood vessels or nerves may result in sexual performance problems.

Next to the prostate are the sphincter muscles that control urination. There are two main sphincter muscles, each of which is made up of fibers arranged in a circular fashion. The internal sphincter surrounds the neck of the bladder. The external sphincter surrounds the urethra at the opening of the prostate. Both of these sphincter muscles work to prevent urine leakage. If both are injured or damaged by surgery or other problems, there may be a loss of urinary control.

THE SIZE OF THE PROSTATE GLAND

During childhood, the prostate gland is not much larger than the eraser on a pencil. During puberty, the prostate rapidly attains the size of a chestnut or a walnut, and develops a pyramidal shape. This change, along with sex organ growth, deepening of the voice, and growth of body hair, is the result of the male hormone testosterone, which is produced in the testicles. Not just the growth of the prostate gland, but also its function, depends on this hormone. (This is one of the reasons that males who for some reason lose their testicles in their youth do not experience the changes of puberty. Their prostates may remain small and without function. And they probably won't experience prostate cancer!)

Following puberty, the prostate reaches normal adult size—approximately two inches by three quarters of an inch by one and a half inches. It then usually remains about the same size until about age fifty, at which point it begins to enlarge. It's not clear why gland enlargement resumes

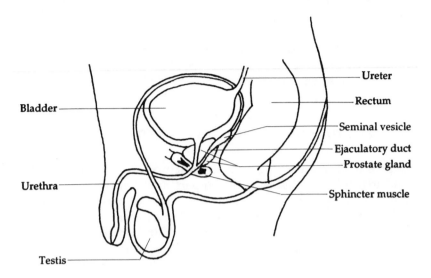

Figure 1.1 The Male Urogenital Tract

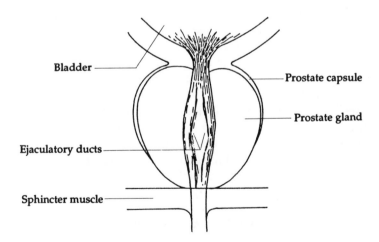

Figure 1.2 The Prostate Gland

at this time, although many researchers believe that it may be a combination of aging and a change in male hormones. This gradual increase in size often results in a condition called *benign prostatic hypertrophy* (BPH), in which the enlargement of the prostate can cause difficulty in urination by pressing on the urethra. BPH eventually affects most men. In fact, prostate problems constitute the bulk of cases seen by urologists.

THE STRUCTURE OF THE PROSTATE GLAND

The prostate is a musculoglandular structure—which means that it's a gland that has muscles. A very compact organ, it contains two major components, an internal zone and an external, or peripheral, zone.

The gland itself is the internal zone. The external or peripheral zone is a dense, fibrous capsule that surrounds the prostate. Visualize the prostate as an orange. There's the meat of the orange (the internal zone), and the outside of the orange, the orange peel (the external or peripheral zone). (See Figure 1.2.) Often, if a prostate gland is surgically removed, it's the internal zone, the gland itself, that is removed from the capsule. However, if surgery is performed for prostate cancer, the capsule is often removed along with the gland.

The prostate is made up of five lobes—two lateral (side), one middle, one anterior (front), and one posterior (back). When the prostate enlarges—as it does in the case of BPH, discussed earlier—the lateral and middle lobes are usually the ones involved. The anterior lobe is a connecting lobe between the lateral lobes, and usually is not involved in this benign condition. The posterior lobe, too, is generally not affected by BPH. However, the posterior lobe often is the location of the beginning of prostate cancer. In fact, it is estimated that 80 to 90 percent of prostate cancers start in this small, flattened lobe.

Inside the prostate, you will find a network of tubular glands that branch out and are imbedded in muscle fibers and connective tissue. During ejaculation, these muscular fibers contract, ejecting the prostatic fluid thorough the prostatic ducts into the urethra, which, as previously discussed, passes through the prostate.

THE FUNCTION OF THE PROSTATE GLAND

It is felt by some that the full function of the prostate is not yet known. However, it is known that the major function of the gland is to assist in sex, or reproduction.

The prostate gland secretes a fluid that forms about 80 percent of the fluid volume of semen. This fluid contains the sperm—although it should be noted that the sperm is produced not in the prostate gland, but in the testicles. The fluid produced by the prostate contains nutrients that enable the sperm to live after ejaculation. The fluid also contains an appropriate degree of acidity for the sperm and allows them to swim actively. This helps the sperm to arrive at and fertilize the female egg. So the prostatic fluid both assists the passage of the sperm and helps to keep the sperm alive.

The prostate gland manufactures this fluid continuously and stores it, awaiting usage. In general, the fluid never runs out. After ejaculation, the glands in the prostate work to replenish the depleted supply.

The prostate is considered to be a gland of external secretion. In other words, it produces a secretion that is discharged only *outside* the body. Because the prostate is an externally secreting gland, the fluid produced by this gland is not considered a hormone. (Hormones, by definition, are secreted in one part of the body in order to start or run an activity in an organ or cells elsewhere in the body.) And so, fortunately, if the prostate is removed, no essential body function is impaired.

As we've already discussed, the testicles, not the prostate, are the primary glands involved in producing the male hormone testosterone—the hormone that causes hair growth, voice deepening, and genital development. The prostate is not involved in any of these functions. However, aside from secreting the prostatic fluid, the prostate also acts as a valve that allows sperm and urine to flow in the proper direction.

DO WOMEN HAVE PROSTATES?

Some experts say that women have prostates that are similar to the glands in a young boy. Research suggests, though, that this tissue, which surrounds the female urethra, may only *look* similar to the male prostate. In general, because both the structure and function of this tissue are different, it is felt that only males have prostate glands that function in the way described in this chapter.

So now you probably know a little bit more about the prostate gland than you did when you first picked this book up. But this book focuses on the condition known as prostate cancer. Let's talk about prostate cancer in more detail.

Chapter 2

WHAT IS
PROSTATE CANCER?

Prostate cancer is just one of the dozens of different types of cancer that can affect us. Before we focus on the unique characteristics of prostate cancer, let's talk a little about cancer in general.

WHAT IS CANCER?

Although you probably have often heard people talk about cancer, you may not have a clear idea of what cancer is. How are cancerous cells different from normal cells? Let's take a look at both normal and cancerous cells, and learn a little more about the nature of cancer.

What Do Normal Cells Do?

All tissues in the body are made up of cells. These cells are the individual building blocks that divide and multiply as needed. Normal cells grow rapidly in infants and children. Then, as the body reaches adult size, cell growth diminishes in speed. This process is so well organized that, in the healthy adult, the normal cells know exactly the right speed at which to grow and divide, and those cells that are born and those that die are approximately equal in number. Certain cells—fingernail and hair cells, for instance—always seem to grow and divide quickly. But most seem to grow and divide frequently only when necessary—for instance, when tissues have been damaged by a wound. After the wound has healed, this accelerated cell growth stops.

Scientists are still trying to understand what controls cell growth. For example, why does a finger or an arm stop growing, rather than growing longer and longer and longer? Some experts believe that cells send out "messages" to each other so that they know exactly when to grow.

What Do Cancer Cells Do?

In cancerous cells, it is felt that the signals used by normal cells are not sent. Somehow, whatever mechanisms control the balance of cell death and cell birth have been damaged or lost. Therefore, cancer cells—mutant, unwanted cells—grow uncontrollably.

Cancer, then, is the uncontrolled growth of mutant cells. The number of these cells exceeds the number of normal cells that die. The cancer cells continue to grow uncontrollably into a tumor, which invades, crowds out, and destroys the healthy tissues around it. This can decrease the amount of cell nourishment received in other normal cells in the body. Body functioning can be affected, which can certainly affect the way you feel physically. And if the growth of these cells is not stopped locally, the cells can spread to other parts of the body. This is the process called *metastasis.*

The rate with which cancer cells divide and grow varies significantly. There are some types of cancers that grow very quickly. There are others that grow very slowly. Fortunately, prostate cancer is most often a slow-growing cancer.

Cancer usually spreads in one of four ways. It can spread via the blood stream, most frequently to the liver, the lungs, and the bones; through the lymphatic system, where it would be found in the lymph nodes; through neighboring tissue; and through open areas in the body, such as the chest cavity or the abdominal cavity.

So the main difference between normal cells and cancer cells is the way they grow. Normal cells grow in a controlled, coordinated way that manages the important functions of the body. Cancer cells act differently. They grow and multiply uncontrollably, increasingly reducing the body's ability to remove them. They have no useful function. They don't help to heal the body, for example. They don't wear out and die as quickly as normal cells do, and while they're alive, they continue to multiply and divide.

Where Do Cancer Cells Come From?

All cells contain genetic material, called DNA. DNA is the material that carries the coded information that tells the cell what to do and how to behave. Any changes or mutations in the genetic material of the cell—any abnormalities in the DNA—can lead to the growth of cancer cells. Because of these changes or mutations, the cells do not respond to the normal controls that maintain proper growth. Thus, cancer cells may no longer be controlled by normal body mechanisms.

What Are the Characteristics of Cancer Cells?

We've just learned how different cancer cells are from normal cells. Although, as you know, there are different types of cancer—which we'll learn about a little later in this chapter—all cancer cells have certain characteristics in common. Let's take a look at the characteristics shared by all cancers.

☐ Cancerous cells tend to develop from a normal cell that has become malignant because of the cell's genetic material, or DNA.

☐ Cancerous cells divide and grow more often and more rapidly than do normal cells.

☐ Unlike normal cells, cancerous cells do not serve a useful function.

☐ Cancerous cells live longer than normal cells live.

☐ Microscopic investigations of cancerous cells show a disordered appearance, as compared with the appearance of normal cells.

☐ While normal cells stay within the region in which they belong, cancerous cells tend to invade tissues in surrounding areas.

☐ Cancerous cells rarely remain even within the surrounding areas. Instead, they often tend to leave the site at which the cancer first developed, and spread to distant parts of the body.

What Are "Precancerous" Cells?

Before we leave the subject of cells, let's take a moment and look at the term "precancerous"—a term you may have heard. Precancerous cells have changed so that they may look abnormal, but are not abnormal enough to be considered cancerous. However, the possibility exists that these abnormal precancerous cells may become cancerous. This doesn't happen to all precancerous cells. Some of them may reverse themselves or be controlled by the immune system.

What Are the Main Categories of Cancer?

There are more than 150 different types of cancer, but the way each cancer grows and spreads is unique. Because of this, diagnosis and treatment of each type of cancer varies in effectiveness and outcome. Unfortunately, neither the course nor the outcome of any particular cancer in any person is predictable. Any time you hear talk of prognosis or outcome, it is based on statistics. There is no way that experts can accurately predict how any one person will respond to treatment.

There are five main categories of cancer. The most common type is the *carcinoma*. Carcinomas are solid tumors that grow in the epithelial tissues, which are the tissues that cover the inside and outside surfaces of all the parts of the body, including the internal organs. A vast majority of all cancers—about 85 percent—are carcinomas. Prostate cancer is an example of a carcinoma, as are breast cancer, lung cancer, colon cancer, intestinal cancer, and skin cancer.

The second type of cancer, the *sarcoma*, develops in bones or connective tissue—tissue that supports or joins other body tissues or parts.

The third type of cancer, *lymphomas*, includes tumors that form in the lymph system, most commonly in the lymph nodes. Hodgkin's disease is a type of lymphoma.

The fourth type, *leukemia*, includes cancers of the circulatory system or the blood. Leukemia usually begins in the blood-forming tissue, bone marrow.

The fifth type, *myelomas*, includes bone-destroying tumors. Myelomas can form at the same time in a number of different places, and occur most often in the ribs, pelvic bones, vertebrae, and flat bones of the skull.

What Are the Main Categories of Tumors?

A tumor is a swelling or enlargement in the body that serves no purpose. It's made up of cells that can be either benign (noncancerous) or malignant (made up of cancer cells). It's important to remember that not every tumor is made up of cancerous cells.

There are three types of cancerous tumors. *Localized tumors* are tumors that remain in the specific site at which they started to grow. Cancerous cells that have moved away from the initial site but remain within one specific area of the body are called *regional tumors*. And cancer cells that have spread to other parts of the body are called *metastasized tumors*.

Some Answers, But Many Questions

There is still much research regarding what causes cancer, what the risk factors are, what the exact mechanism is that causes cancer cells to grow uncontrollably, and how cancer treatment and outcome can be improved. However, one essential thing to remember is that cancer is not contagious. One person does not "catch" cancer from another person.

There is also no evidence that cancer is caused by injury. Sometimes people are afraid that an injury may damage certain cells, leading to the formation of cancer cells. However, there is no evidence suggesting that injury leads to the development of cancerous tumors.

It is felt that cancerous cells may be present in our bodies all the time, and that our immune system is normally able to maintain a system of "checks and balances" and keep control over the undesired growth of these abnormal cells. However, there are times when our immune system is unable to function effectively. What happens then? The cancerous cells may grow unchecked and become a cancer.

Much research is now focusing on why the immune system is sometimes not able to control the growth of cancer cells. For example, one theory is that cancer cells secrete some kind of chemical that decreases the effectiveness of the immune system. Cancer cells then grow so rapidly that the immune system is just not able to keep up.

The goal of cancer treatment, of course, is to eliminate these cancer cells. Some of the modern treatments used to accomplish this include surgery, chemotherapy, radiation therapy, and hormone therapy. There are also a number of newer methods that are being investigated, including nutritional therapy and heat and cold therapy.

Occasionally, cancer cells seem to disappear by themselves. This is called *spontaneous remission*. Although it's not completely understood why this sometimes occurs, one theory is that the body's immune system is somehow able to regain sufficient strength to control or eliminate these cells. This is one of the reasons for the development of a new type of treatment, called immunotherapy, designed to strengthen the immune system so that it can regain its controlling role.

WHAT IS PROSTATE CANCER?

Prostate cancer is the most serious problem that can develop with the prostate. However, early detection and diagnosis and prompt effective treatment can be successful in curing, or at least controlling, this disorder.

This may sound strange, but prostate cancer is one of the best cancers you can get. Why? Because prostate cancer is usually very slow-growing. If treatment at an early stage is not able to cure it, there are a number of other techniques that can suppress the cancer and help you to live a long, healthy, and productive life. In fact, many men with prostate cancer aren't even aware of its existence. In many cases, prostate cancer is noticed only after a person has died from a disorder unrelated to the prostate. You should be aware, though, that prostate cancer is not always slow-growing. In some cases, prostate cancer can be virulent—

although it should be noted that doctors have no way of determining how active the prostate cancer will be.

As discussed in Chapter 1, researchers have estimated that 80 to 90 percent of prostate cancers begin at the back of the prostate, in the posterior lobe. Generally, the cancer starts in the epithelial cells, which are the cells that line the outside of the gland. (Remember the peel of the orange?) Often, the surface where the cancer begins is the one that borders the rectum. As you'll learn in Chapter 3, this location is very helpful for early diagnosis.

Because prostate cancer usually starts far away from the urethra, very few symptoms—such as difficulty in urinating—may be noticed for a long time. That's why this is considered to be a "silent cancer." There are no other warning signals that arise during the early stages either.

Prostate cancer spreads through the gland like slow-moving lava. As the tumor enlarges, it hardens. Eventually, the cancer can obstruct the flow of urine from the bladder. How? As the tumor grows, moving toward the front of the gland, it shuts off the urethra. In more advanced cases, the cancer breaks away from its confinement within the prostate and spreads to other parts of the body.

Who Gets Prostate Cancer?

What is known about how many people get prostate cancer? Prostate cancer was a relatively rare disorder before 1900. Today, it is considered the second most common male cancer. Ranking only behind lung cancer, prostate cancer accounts for approximately 18 percent of all cancer in males.

Prostate cancer is definitely age-related, being the most common cancer in men over the age of fifty. Approximately 80 percent of men diagnosed with prostate cancer are over age sixty-five when a tumor in the prostate is first detected. The average age of men at the time they are diagnosed with prostate cancer is seventy-three. It is, in fact, relatively uncommon in younger men, with only 2 percent of all prostate cancers occurring in men under the age of fifty.

Prostate cancer can occur in all races and ethnic groups. However, its incidence is relatively low in the Near East, in parts of Africa and South America, and in China, Japan, and the Philippines. It is far more common in North American and European men. And the highest incidence of prostate cancer in the world seems to be among African-American men, whose risk of prostate cancer is 40 percent higher than that of whites. Also, prostate cancer tends to occur more among married men than among men who are single.

It has been estimated that approximately 60,000 to 90,000 cases of prostate cancer are diagnosed each year in the United States alone. In fact, the disease is so prevalent that, by age eighty, it is thought that almost all men have microscopic prostate cancers. However, as previously discussed, in many cases it is not diagnosed.

The number of people being diagnosed with prostate cancer is increasing. This is partly because people are now more health conscious than ever before, and are seeing their doctors more often. In addition, doctors are now better able to identify prostate cancer. There has been much improvement in diagnostic testing, and there is also a greater awareness of the condition. The number of cases is also increasing because men are now living to later and later ages.

What Causes Prostate Cancer?

Why does prostate cancer occur? Why do some people experience more problems with their prostate than others? Researchers continue to search for answers to these and other questions.

The exact cause of prostate cancer is still not clearly understood. The leading hypotheses target hormonal, dietary, and genetic factors. Let's briefly discuss these three areas of investigation.

Much prostate cancer research focuses on hormonal imbalances. Men produce both male and female hormones. It is known that male hormones can speed up the growth of prostate cancer, while female hormones can shrink the tumor or, at least, slow its growth. Some researchers have speculated that changes in the relative amounts of these hormones may be involved in the development of prostate cancer. The fact that men who have had their testicles removed before the onset of puberty almost never get prostate cancer also suggests that a hormonal factor may bring about cancerous changes in the gland.

Some researchers think that diet—especially one that is high in fat— may play a role in the development of prostate cancer. Why? There is a higher incidence of prostate cancer, for example, in Japanese men who have migrated to America than in Japanese men who still live in Japan. It has been hypothesized that the main difference between these two groups may be the high-fat diet more prevalent in the United States. In addition, dietary factors may play a role in the high incidence of prostate cancer among African-Americans, who, it has been suggested, often eat diets that are higher in fat than the diets of other Americans. Some studies have indicated that individuals who consistently follow low-cholesterol diets, diets rich in green or yellow vegetables, or vegetarian diets, have a lower-than-average incidence of prostate cancer.

The fact that in some cases prostate cancer seems to run in families is also under investigation. There is still no clear evidence indicating whether genetic tendencies play a part in prostate cancer. It may be that family tendencies to develop prostate cancer involve environmental factors, or that the prevalence of such tendencies within a family may simply be a coincidence.

One factor frustrating researchers trying to identify causes of prostate cancer is the fact that prostate cancer exists almost exclusively in human beings. As a result, the researchers have been unable to do any kind of meaningful research with animals. So, unfortunately, the causes of prostate cancer are still unknown. On the other hand, contrary to past beliefs, we do now know that prostate disease is not caused by venereal disease, tobacco use, excessive weight gain, alcohol use, masturbation, or frequent sexual activity. And, even though we don't yet know the cause of prostate cancer, researchers are constantly developing better diagnostic and treatment techniques.

What Are the Symptoms of Prostate Cancer?

Unfortunately, there are often no signs or symptoms of prostate cancer, especially in the early stages. In fact, prostate cancer can grow for quite a while before any noticeable symptoms appear. (Years ago, the diagnosis of prostate cancer was most often made after it had spread to the bones, as this would start causing bone pain.) Any symptoms that do occur are usually similar to the symptoms of benign prostatic hypertrophy (BPH), a disorder in which the prostate becomes swollen and presses on the urethra, causing obstruction and, possibly, difficulty or discomfort during urination. But, as mentioned earlier, a large percentage of prostate cancers begin near the posterior, or outer back, part of the gland. In these cases, the cancer may not create irritative or obstructive symptoms until it has developed sufficiently to affect most of the gland. Then, and only then, would there be any symptoms.

As the tumor develops, most or all of the prostate hardens and becomes nodular in appearance. In fact, because of the pressure placed on the urethra, it may become virtually impossible to insert a catheter—a flexible tube used to drain fluids—or a cystoscope—a diagnostic tool used to examine the urinary tract and aid in the removal of tumors and other growths. Eventually, the pressure placed on the urethra by the enlarged prostate may lead to symptoms of irritation—including the urgent need to urinate frequently, nocturia (urination at night), and dysuria (painful urination)—and symptoms of obstruction—hesitant urination (a urinary stream that is weak or interrupted) and a feeling that the bladder has not been completely emptied. Other symptoms that may be experienced include kidney pain or infection due to obstruction, pain in the lower back or pelvic area (for this to be a legitimate symptom, it should last for more than two weeks), loss of appetite, fatigue, weight loss, weakness in the legs, incontinence (the inability to control urination), and blood in the urine. But if you experience any of these symptoms, check them out before you jump to any frightening conclusions!

How Does Prostate Cancer Metastasize?

As the malignant cancer cells spread throughout the prostate, most or all of the prostate gland becomes hardened with the cancer. Prostate cancer, like most other cancers, is then likely to metastasize, or spread to other parts of the body, if left untreated. Sometimes, prostate cancer may be so slow-growing that nothing appears to change. But in other cases it may spread to adjacent tissues and involve the seminal vesicles—the saclike glands that lie behind the bladder and release a fluid that forms part of the semen. The cancer cells may then spread through the blood and lymph vessels, and then cause new colonies of cells or new tumors to grow in other locations. Most commonly, prostate cancer spreads into the lymph nodes and to bones in the pelvic area and lower spine, but it may also spread to many other parts of the body, including the ribs, skull, and other bones, the liver, and the lungs.

What Is the Prognosis?

So what are the chances for successfully treating prostate cancer? The answer really depends on whom you ask and what you read. Some information suggests that the chance for a successful outcome is high—much higher than that for lung cancer and other common cancers. This doesn't mean that the prostate cancer will necessarily be cured. However, in most cases, it is one of the slowest growing of all cancers. In addition, because so many men with prostate cancer are older—in many cases, more than sixty-five years of age—some other disorder is usually the cause of death. So the vast majority of individuals with prostate cancer do not die of this disease. In fact, studies indicate that, despite the prevalence of prostate cancer, only 2.5 percent of all men will ultimately die of this disorder.

Other information suggests that the chances for a successful outcome are not good, simply because most of the medical efforts focus only on delaying the growth of the disease. So you may read in the newspaper about famous people who are dying of prostate cancer. And you may read that approximately 35,000 men each year die of prostate cancer. But these reports should say that approximately this number of men die *with* prostate cancer—meaning that these men have prostate cancer, but that it is not necessarily the cause of death.

This is not to say, though, that prostate cancer is not life-threatening. It can be. But that doesn't mean that it will be life-threatening in your case. That's why you're reading this book, to try to learn everything you can about living successfully despite prostate cancer. If you have prostate cancer, focus your energy on constructively fighting the disease. Every effort you put into taking care of yourself will be a major step in the right direction.

Chapter 3

HOW IS PROSTATE CANCER DIAGNOSED?

After Jack got over his initial shock at being diagnosed with prostate cancer, he asked his doctor to explain how he had pinpointed the problem. Jack's doctor then told him about the procedures physicians use to accurately diagnose prostate cancer. He explained to Jack that early diagnosis is essential because the earlier the cancer is caught, the better the chance for successful treatment.

So how do physicians determine if someone has prostate cancer? The diagnosis of prostate cancer is made as a result of the patient's medical history, a detailed physical examination, and an assessment of appropriate laboratory test results.

The procedures used for prostate cancer diagnosis fall into four general categories: digital rectal examination, blood tests, visualization techniques, and tissue examination (biopsy). Let's take a look at each of these categories, learn about the purpose and limitations of each test, and see how each can contribute to an accurate diagnosis.

THE DIGITAL RECTAL EXAMINATION (DRE)

The first step in diagnosing prostate cancer is the physical examination. Because the prostate is located right next to the rectum and about one and a half inches from the anal opening, it is relatively easy to reach it with a finger or an instrument. And, as discussed in Chapters 1 and 2, most cancers begin in the posterior, or back, lobe of the prostate, near the rectum. As a result, a digital (using the finger) rectal examination (DRE), performed during a routine physical examination, can often detect a tumor in the prostate gland even before symptoms develop.

The physician examines the prostate by inserting a gloved finger into the rectum and pressing toward the pubic bone to feel the posterior lobe of the prostate. The normal prostate has a smooth surface and an elastic consistency. A cancerous tumor, however, creates a small, hard area, or nodule. As the cancer develops, this hard nodule becomes larger, and more nodules may appear. So the doctor examines the size and consistency of the prostate, and feels for any hard bumps or nodules, which may be either raised or imbedded in the prostate tissue.

Although a DRE can't always guarantee early detection of prostate cancer, it still is a very effective procedure. In fact, it is considered so important that the American Cancer Society recommends that all men over the age of forty get an annual DRE. Most experts emphatically state that if more men had regular digital rectal examinations, more early cancers would be detected and cured before they spread.

Limitations of the DRE

One problem involved in the diagnosis of prostate cancer is that not all hard areas in the prostate are cancerous. In fact, experience suggests that only about half of the nodules that physicians notice during examinations are cancerous. Other hard objects may be stones or signs of chronic infection. So whenever a hard area is felt during the DRE, further testing is done. Normally, the next step is a trip to the urologist for further diagnosis and treatment.

It is also possible—although unlikely—that the DRE will indicate that the prostate is fine when cancer is actually present. There are four ways in which this mistake may occur:

1. The cancer nodule may be located far enough away from the rectum to escape detection during the DRE. For example, it might develop in the anterior, or front, lobe—although this location is fairly uncommon.
2. The nodule may be cushioned by the prostate enlargement common in benign prostatic hypertrophy (BPH), making it virtually impossible to detect the cancer through touch. (See page 6 for more about BPH.)
3. The cancer nodule may be so tiny that it can't be felt at all.
4. On infrequent occasions, the cancer cells may not form a distinct, palpable nodule.

As you see, the DRE is not foolproof. But even though it has its limitations, the DRE is still one of the best means we have of detecting prosate cancer in its earliest and most curable stage.

BLOOD TESTS

The two blood tests most commonly used to detect prostate cancer are the prostate-specific antigen test, and the prostatic acid phosphatase test. These tests are often performed prior to the biospy when prostate cancer is suspected. Let's see how each of these tests can contribute to an accurate diagnosis.

The Prostate-Specific Antigen (PSA) Blood Test

This test is often used to detect or confirm the existence of BPH or prostate cancer, and has been helpful in diagnosing prostate cancers more quickly.

Prostate-specific antigen (PSA) is a substance that is normally produced in the prostate. Enlargement of the prostate may result in slightly elevated levels of this antigen simply because there is more prostate to make more antigen! When cancerous cells exist in the prostate and spread to other parts of the body, they, too, produce PSA. And cancerous prostate tissue makes about ten times as much of the substance as normal cells do. Blood tests can be used to detect higher levels of PSA in the blood stream. The higher the level, the more likely it is that the cancer has spread to other parts of the body.

To avoid false positive results, this test should not be performed for forty-eight to seventy-two hours after a rectal examination. The reason for this is that DREs can result in the release of additional prostate-specific antigen, bringing about a false positive finding. Another factor that can inflate PSA readings is infection of the prostate. Nevertheless, the PSA test is considered so valuable that in fall of 1992, the American Cancer Society recommended that annual PSA testing start at age fifty for all men, and that it begin at age forty for men at high risk—those with a family history of the disorder, and all African-Americans. And many feel that the most thorough approach would be to use both a rectal exam and a PSA test.

The Prostatic Acid Phosphatase (PAP) Blood Test

Like PSA, prostatic acid phosphatase (PAP), an enzyme, is normally produced in the prostate gland, and continues to be manufactured even when the prostate cells become cancerous. When cancerous cells break through the prostatic capsule and spread to other parts of the body, they continue producing the enzyme, eventually leading to higher levels of PAP in the blood. So elevated levels of PAP, detected through a blood test, may suggest that the cancer has spread to the lymph nodes or other parts of the body.

Like the prostate-specific antigen test, this test may give a false postive result if performed within seventy-two hours following a rectal examination. And also like the PSA test, the PAP test may indicate benign prostatic hypertrophy, rather than prostate cancer.

VISUALIZATION TECHNIQUES

A number of visualization techniques—techniques used to provide a visual image of structures inside the body—are often an important part of the diagnostic process. These tests can help the doctor determine whether or not the tumor is still localized.

In deciding which of these tests should be used in your case, your doctor will take your age, your overall health, and a number of other factors into consideration. Let's briefly discuss some of the more commonly used methods of visualization.

Scans and X-Rays

Bone scans—and, occasionally, specific bone x-rays—may be performed to see if the prostate cancer has spread to the bones, the most common site of prostate cancer metastasis. Chest x-rays may be performed to see if the cancer has spread to the lungs.

Computerized Tomography (CT) Scan and Magnetic Resonance Imaging (MRI)

Both computerized tomography (CT) scans and magnetic resonance imaging (MRI) are used to determine the stage of the cancer. (See page 24 for information on staging.) In the diagnosis of prostate cancer, abdominal CT scans and MRIs look specifically at the lymph nodes and the liver.

The CT scan, also called a CAT scan, produces a cross-sectional view of an organ of the body. How does it work? In this hour-long procedure, you lie on a table that moves through a tunnel. While in the tunnel, a radioactive beam rotates fully around your body in a 360-degree arc. Information from this beam is fed into a computer and is translated into tiny dots of varying density, which appear first on a screen and then on x-ray film. Sometimes, in order to make the images of the structures even sharper, you may be asked to drink a dye, or you may receive an intravenous injection of a dye.

The MRI is a recently developed diagnostic technique that makes use of a magnetic field and radio frequency signals instead of the radiation used in CT scans. As with the CT scan, during this hour-long procedure you move through a tunnel, and cross-sectional pictures of organs and tissues appear first on a screen, and later on x-ray film.

Although they are not 100-percent accurate, both CT scans and MRIs are helpful in evaluating prostate cancer, especially when determining if the cancer has spread to lymph nodes, if the lymph nodes are enlarged, or if the cancer has spread to other parts of the body, such as the bones, lungs, or liver.

The Cystoscope

The cystoscope is an instrument used to examine the urethra and bladder so that the physician can determine if the tumor is pressing on the urethra and if the cancer has spread into the bladder.

The cystoscope looks something like a skinny periscope. The instrument has two very thin tubes. One is used to introduce fluids into the area being examined (the fluid is inserted and then released), and the other contains the light and lenses that allow the physician to see the structures.

Cystoscope exams usually take one to two minutes. The lubricated shaft of the cystoscope is inserted gently through the urethra. During the insertion process, the physician can see the walls of the urethra and can determine if there has been any narrowing of the urethra due to prostatic enlargement. Although the cystoscope is used primarily to examine the inside of the bladder, the ease of insertion lets the doctor know whether there are prostate problems, since the instrument cannot pass through the urethra if the prostate is exerting too much pressure on it. (As you might remember, the urethra passes through the middle of the gland.)

The Intravenous Pyelogram (IVP)

The intravenous pyelogram (IVP)—also called a urogram—is an x-ray used to evaluate the prostate and bladder. Specifically, the IVP shows what effect, if any, the prostate cancer has had on the bladder and the ureters (the tubes that carry urine from the kidneys to the bladder), including the cancer's effect on bladder emptying.

During this procedure, a colorless fluid—an organic iodine solution that, like bone, shows as a white area on x-ray film—is injected into a vein in the arm. Like any waste product, this dye is filtered out of the blood by the kidneys, at which point x-rays can pick up the urinary tract and show outlines of the interior of the bladder, the kidneys, and the ureters.

Ultrasound

Ultrasound imaging—sometimes called sonograms—is often used to establish the size, shape, and location of the prostate gland, as well as to determine if there are any abnormalities in the structures being examined. Ultrasound is also helpful in guiding the movement of the needle when a biopsy is performed.

During this procedure, high-frequency sound waves are aimed at the part of the body being examined. Because these sound waves pass through tissues of different densities at different rates, the outlines of organs or tumors can be seen, and an image can be recorded.

In the diagnosis of prostate cancer, a type of ultrasound called transrectal ultrasound may be used. For this ten-to-twenty-minute procedure, a probe covered with a water-filled balloon is inserted in the rectum. The probe both produces sound waves and receives echoes from the waves. These echoes are electronically processed to create a fairly detailed picture first on a screen, and later on film.

Some experts feel that transrectal ultrasound can be even more effective in pinpointing the location of cancerous tumors than can the digital rectal examination (DRE). In some cases, in fact, this procedure has been useful in finding tumors missed during DREs. However, the fact that there may be either false positive or false negative readings is cause for concern.

At this time, researchers are modifying ultrasound machines to use a type of sound wave called doppler. The aim of this research is to more efficiently pick up malignancies.

PROSTATE BIOPSY

The biopsy is a minor surgical procedure that involves taking a small piece of tissue or group of cells from the area being evaluated. This procedure is performed by a urologist to determine if there are any cancerous cells in the area.

For many years, the most common biopsy method made use of a special needle, which was inserted through the rectum so that a small piece of tissue could be obtained from the area in question. This procedure took approximately ten minutes, and was mildly uncomfortable, although usually no anesthesia was used. Now, virtually all doctors use a spring-loaded biopsy gun, often assisted by ultrasound, to perform this tissue biopsy. The spring-loaded gun takes the same kind of sample as that removed by the needle, but in this case, the procedure is relatively painless. Both the needle and gun biopsies are considered to be most accurate in diagnosing more advanced cancers, as in these cases, there are larger nodules. When the nodules are very small, it may be quite difficult to find the area and obtain a sample.

A recently developed biopsy procedure, which decreases bleeding as well as the chance of infection, is now being used by some urologists. It's called fine-needle aspiration cytology. During this procedure, a very fine needle is inserted in the patient's rectum, and, using suction—or aspiration—cells are removed from approximately four different spots in the prostate. This is considered to be a quick, safe, and excellent diagnostic procedure that is relatively painless—no anesthesia is needed, and the procedure often takes no more than two or three minutes. If the results are uncertain, the procedure may be repeated, or a more traditional biopsy of the prostate may be performed to get a larger sample of tissue.

Regardless of which procedure is used, if the biopsy indicates cancer, additional tests will be conducted to determine the extent of the cancer so that appropriate treatment can be chosen. If the biopsy is negative—if it shows no cancer cells—but the doctor still suspects a problem, the procedure may be repeated in a few months.

OTHER DIAGNOSTIC PROCEDURES

Other screening or diagnostic tests may also be performed—often, to rule out various problems. For example, urinalysis is used to determine whether or not there is an infection or blood in the urine. Blood tests other than the PSA and PAP are done to more fully evaluate blood chemistry. Liver function may also be tested, since prostate cancer can spread to this organ.

If your doctor suspects that the prostate cancer has spread to the lymph nodes, but this has not been confirmed, he or she may use a procedure called pelvic lymph node dissection—a procedure performed during prostatectomy surgery. (For more information on this surgery, see Chapter 5.) Sometimes, even though a CT scan or MRI shows no lymph node involvement, this procedure reveals tiny cancer cells in the lymph nodes. This then changes the stage of the cancer—something you'll learn about in the following discussion.

STAGING

When prostate cancer is diagnosed, the tumors that are discovered vary widely in terms of how they look, how different they are from normal cells (differentiation), how fast they grow (aggressiveness), and how much they have spread (invasiveness). These are all important factors, but in determining the stage of the prostate cancer—an essential step in choosing treatment—only invasiveness is involved. So the tests described throughout this chapter are performed to determine whether the cancer is contained, has spread locally, or has spread to distant parts of the body. Let's look at the four stages of prostate cancer, and see what each stage means in terms of treatment.

Stage A

In Stage A, there are no symptoms at all, and a rectal examination may suggest that the prostate is normal. If surgery happens to be performed for benign prostatic hypertrophy, however, cancerous cells may be found in the prostate.

Stage A has two subcategories. In Substage A1, one or two small areas of cancer can be found within the prostate. In this stage, even with no treatment, there is a very good chance for survival to normal life expectancy. In Substage A2, cancer can be found in more than a few places within the prostate. Treatment is usually required in this case. Depending on a number of factors—including the person's age and overall health, the aggressiveness of the tumor, and, of course, the person's wishes—this treatment may include surgical removal of the prostate gland (prostatectomy) and/or radiation.

Stage B

In Stage B, the tumors, still totally within the gland, can often be felt during a digital rectal examination. But there still may be no noticeable symptoms.

Stage B has two subcategories. In the first, B1, tumors are growing in only one lobe of the prostate, and a small, discrete nodule, usually less than a half inch in size, can be found. In Substage B2, nodules have invaded more than one lobe of the prostate.

Because it is more likely that Substage B2 cancers will spread beyond the prostate—and even some B1 tumors can spread—surgery is usually prescribed in Stage B. However, depending on a number of factors, radiation therapy may be used along with or instead of surgery.

Stage C

Stage C, like Stages A and B, has two substages. In Substage C1, cancerous tumors have spread outside the gland. In Substage C2, tumors may have invaded the seminal vesicles or the neck of the bladder. Research suggests that C2 tumors have a greater chance of spreading to the pelvic lymph nodes than do C1 tumors.

Because the entire prostate may be cancerous in Stage C, this is the stage in which patients often begin to experience problems with urination. Depending on various factors, surgery, radiation, or hormone therapy may be prescribed during this stage.

Stage D

In this stage, cancer has spread beyond the prostatic capsule itself, invading the lymph nodes and, possibly, other parts of the body.

In Substage D1, the prostate cancer has spread only to the lymph nodes. In D2, the cancer has metastasized beyond the immediate area, and can be found in other organs, such as the bones and the lungs. As a result, individuals with Stage D prostate cancer often suffer from urinary difficulty and experience back pain, weight loss, and blood in the urine. Yet there are many people in Stage D who experience no symptoms at all.

While Stage A, B, and C cancers are considered to be potentially curable, Stage D cancers are often considered to be incurable, but can often be easily controlled. So the goal of treatment is to suppress symptoms and perpetuate life, usually through the use of radiation or hormone therapy.

When looking at the staging of prostate cancer, it's important to keep in mind that cancer does not necessarily move from one stage to the next in order. For example, there may be times when a tumor in the Stage A classification immediately moves to advanced metastatic disease.

As stated earlier, the staging of prostate cancer is an essential part of the decision-making process regarding treatment. In the next few chapters, we'll talk about the various types of treatment that are available for prostate cancer.

PART II

THE TREATMENT
OF PROSTATE CANCER

Chapter 4

THE TREATMENT OF PROSTATE CANCER— AN INTRODUCTION

So far, we have discussed many things about prostate cancer, including what it is, who is most likely to get it, what some of the symptoms are, and how it may be diagnosed. These things are all very important, but what's the most important thing? Yes, what can be done to get rid of, or at least control, your cancer! True? Fortunately, the development of successful treatments for prostate cancer has made its prognosis quite hopeful.

You probably have some important questions. What will your doctors do? What will your doctors tell you to do? What is the treatment for your prostate cancer and how will it affect you? How can you control any physical consequences, either of the cancer itself or of your treatment? How can you help yourself get back into the mainstream of life? Let's begin by answering some of the questions you may have about the treatment of prostate cancer.

WHAT IS YOUR ROLE IN TREATMENT?

There are always things you can do to help yourself. It doesn't matter how much medical knowledge you have—or don't have. Physicians can provide much in the way of medical information, treatment, and expertise. And family and friends can provide emotional support, caring, and guidance. But you are the only one who can make the many decisions necessary to organize your life as helpfully as possible. These decisions may be small, but they will be critical in determining how prostate cancer affects you. It is obvious that you can play an important role in influencing the way you feel. But that's not enough. No single factor is enough. To help yourself best, a whole-package approach is essential—an approach that enables you to help yourself in as many ways as possible, both medically and psychologically.

WHAT IS THE GOAL OF TREATMENT?

In part, the goal of prostate cancer treatment is to do the best possible job of keeping your health intact—to cure, or at least suppress, the disease. In addition, your treatment should reduce the symptoms themselves, reduce any impact the symptoms may have on your life, and strengthen your body.

WHAT ARE THE COMPONENTS OF TREATMENT PROGRAMS?

All treatment programs should involve a number of components, including both the prescribed medical treatment itself and a comprehensive program of stress management, exercise, nutrition, and psychological improvement. This chapter will provide an overview of these different components. More details about all of them will be found later in the book.

The Medical Components of Treatment

Once prostate cancer has been diagnosed, the next step is to find out whether or not the cancer has spread to other parts of the body. If the cancer is confined to the prostate, your doctors will focus on which type of treatment can best deal with this. If the cancer has spread outside the prostate to the seminal vesicles, lymph nodes, or bones, a different type of treatment will be considered. Keep in mind that most treatment efforts are made up of both curative measures—measures that aim to cure the disease or stop its spread—and palliative measures—measures that aim to increase your level of comfort.

Treatment is often dependent on the virulence of the cancer itself. This makes it difficult for doctors to determine what treatment will be best, simply because, as discussed in Chapter 2, there is no way of predicting how virulent or active the prostate cancer will be. The choice of treatment often depends on a number of other factors, too, including your age, your general health, and the preference of the professionals you're working with. Is that all? No, other factors may include your family situation, your occupation, and, of course, your own feelings and preferences!

This makes it sound like there are lots of different treatments for prostate cancer. That's not really true. The most commonly used treatment methods include watchful waiting, surgery, radiation, and hormone therapy. Chemotherapy, other than hormone therapy, is rarely used.

Treatment for Localized Cancer

If, as a result of all of the careful diagnostic procedures, it is determined that the cancer is still localized and contained within the prostate—in other words, that the cancer is in Stage A or B—the aim of treatment is usually to eliminate the cancer and effect a cure. This is most often done with surgery—the radical prostatectomy, in which the entire prostate gland and capsule are removed. (See Chapter 5 for information about the radical prostatectomy.) Either external radiation treatments or radiation implants, in which radioactive seeds or pellets are implanted in the prostate, may also be used to eliminate whatever tumor still exists. (See Chapter 6 for information on radiation treatments.)

Sometimes, if you feel well and your cancer is at an early stage, the standard approach is often just to wait and see what happens. There also may be times when treatment can be postponed, especially if the tumor has not spread beyond the gland itself. Decisions of this type are sometimes a reflection of the patient's age. Younger men without metastases may opt for a more aggressive treatment. Because the cancer usually grows so slowly, older men may opt to have no treatment. Often, a wait-and-see approach includes repetitions of the prostate-specific antigen (PSA) test every few months or so to make sure that there have been no significant changes.

If aggressive treatment is indicated, there is no definitive answer as to which procedure—radiation therapy or surgery—is more likely to be curative for localized prostatic cancer. The survival rates for both treatments are estimated to be the same. So, what should you do? There is rarely a clear choice. Of course, most urologists have their own preference regarding procedures. Make sure you fully understand what their choice is, and what their rationale is for using it. Keep in mind, though, that some studies have suggested that surgery or radiation therapy may not be better than watchful waiting when prostate cancer is in its early stages. The best course of action is to discuss your options with your doctor, and decide on a treatment together.

Treatment for Metastasized Cancer

If diagnostic tests suggest that the cancer has spread beyond the prostate—that the cancer is in Stage C or D—cure may no longer be the goal of treatment. Rather, control will be the immediate goal—slowing down the growth of the tumor, relieving any pain, and avoiding obstructions to the urethra.

While the surgical removal of affected tissues is sometimes used in cases of metastasized prostate cancer, radiation and hormone therapy are by far the most common treatments. In Stage C, radiation is often the treatment of choice, although hormone therapy may be used instead of or in addition to the radiation. In Stage D, hormone therapy is used with greater frequency. Again, though, radiation may be preferred in some cases, or the two techniques may be used together. (See Chapter 7 for information on hormone therapy.)

Other Treatments

Two other prostate cancer treatments are now occasionally used, or may be used in the future. Because these treatments do not now play an important part in prostate cancer therapy, we will not provide detailed discussions of them later in the book. Here, though, is a brief glimpse of chemotherapy and cryosurgery.

Chemotherapy involves the use of drugs to treat disease. These drugs work in two different ways. Some of them stop DNA formation and, as a result, make it impossible for cancer cells to divide and multiply. Other drugs work by paralyzing the cancer cells when they're in the middle of the division process.

Chemotherapy is not often used for prostate cancer. However, if hormone therapy does not work to slow or stop cancer growth, chemotherapy drugs may be prescribed in an attempt to slow the growth and relieve symptoms. Once prostate cancer has become widespread, though, chemotherapy has been found to be beneficial for only 20 percent or so of the individuals who try it.

Cryosurgery, which is treatment by freezing, involves the insertion of a probe into the prostate. The probe is then cooled to subfreezing temperatures through the use of liquid nitrogen, freezing and destroying the cancer cells. Although cryosurgery may become an important method of treating prostate cancer in the future, at present, it is still in the experimental stages. However, cryosurgery has already become an effective tool in the treatment of many other cancers, as well as in the treatment of skin disorders.

Because you might receive different treatments at different times, it is important to be aware of all of the different types of treatment available for prostate cancer. In your particular case, there may be very little choice regarding the treatment available to you. However, if your situation does allow you to make a choice, you'll want to get all the information you need to make the best possible decision. Keep in mind that there is no consensus among experts regarding the best treatment for prostate cancer. To determine which course of action is right for you, you'll want to listen to the recommendation of your doctor, and also to find out what the advantages and disadvantages of each treatment are, what the side effects might be, and what the survival rates are.

Informed Consent

Throughout your treatment for prostate cancer, it's important to remain aware of the rights of "informed consent." What is informed consent? It is written permission, obtained from a patient, to perform certain tests or procedures. Informed consent came to be because of increases in the number of malpractice claims. The goal is for both physicians and patients to feel more comfortable, knowing that detailed information has been presented and discussed about the prescribed procedure, and that, aware of the possible risks, the patient has given his consent.

Why is informed consent so important in cancer treatment? First, many different types of treatment for cancer are experimental. Therefore, it is important to know what types of treatment you are receiving, whether or not they are experimental, and what may occur as a result of their use. Second, even though diagnostic procedures have improved significantly in recent years, there is still no way that doctors can be absolutely sure what is going on inside of your body until they get in there and look! If you're having surgery, and it is performed under general anesthesia, you'll be unconscious during the operation. Doctors have to know that they can go ahead and do whatever is medically correct without first waking you up and asking for your approval.

Informed consent has five primary elements:

1. An explanation of the treatment being proposed.
2. An explanation of the possible risks, as well as the possible benefits, of that treatment.
3. An explanation of the possible alternatives to that treatment.
4. Plenty of time for you to ask any questions you may have.
5. The option for you to withdraw—at any time—from any research or experimental treatments you may be undergoing.

It is inappropriate for informed consent procedures to replace doctor-patient communication. Rather, you should think of these procedures as a springboard for additional effective communication between you and your doctor.

The Nonmedical Components of Treatment

In addition to medical treatment, there are a number of other ways you can help yourself. Stress management, exercise, proper nutrition, and various coping strategies can go a long way in improving both your physical and your emotional well-being.

Stress Management

Stress management is an important part of your program for dealing with prostate cancer. It includes a number of different strategies, dealing with both physiological and psychological stress. An important goal in stress management is to improve your feeling of being in control, in terms of both your emotions and your behavior. (See Chapter 15 for more information on stress.)

Exercise

Exercise is also an important part of your treatment package. Exercise can help you feel better physically, as well as reduce stress and enhance self-esteem. It can also be very helpful in improving the way you perceive your health.

Although some people with prostate cancer may have been told to avoid or minimize physical exertion, it has been found that a gradually increasing program of physical exercise is often helpful in the treatment of this disorder. Of course, all exercise should be done only under strict medical supervision. (See Chapter 22 for more information on exercise.)

Diet

Proper diet is an important part of any treatment program. It's necessary to nourish your body and maintain as much strength and vitality as you can. In fact, many experts believe that diet plays an essential role in the treatment of cancer. And you want to do everything you can to help yourself, right? (See Chapter 21 for more information on diet.)

Psychological Improvement

An important component of treatment programs for prostate cancer is successful coping—effectively dealing with the ups and downs of your cancer experience, and maintaining a positive mental attitude. There are many practical things that can be done to improve your mental attitude, and we'll be talking about a number of them in more detail later in the book.

EACH PERSON IS UNIQUE

Your experience with prostate cancer is unique. As a result, your physician will set up a treatment program based specifically on your needs. It is very important for you to feel at ease with your physician. You should have confidence in the treatment program prescribed for you. Whom should you be working with? Often the most important professionals in the treatment of prostate cancer are a well-trained board-certified urologist and a radiation oncologist. Other specialists may be involved as well. (See Chapter 29 for information on choosing and establishing good relationships with physicians.)

Imagine this. You hear of somebody else with prostate cancer receiving different treatment from a different physician. You start to believe that the other treatment program might be better. You start losing confidence first in your treatment plan, and then in your own physician. Not a great feeling, is it? Remember that there is no one answer! What works for somebody else will not necessarily work for you. *But* you should always feel free to discuss these feelings with your doctor. Don't let your concerns simmer inside you!

Remember that regardless of the support that you receive from the people around you—including family, friends, and professionals—you are the person who is ultimately responsible for doing the best you can to take care of yourself. You are the person who can make the necessary changes, work to improve your positive attitude, and deal as productively as you can with the condition.

MOVING ON . . .

Professionals involved in the treatment of prostate cancer recognize that the best, most effective treatment program incorporates proper medical treatment or intervention, as prescribed; strategies for coping with emotional reactions; and the adjustment of general lifestyle, including any changes in activity necessitated by your condition, as well as attention to nutritional needs and proper exercise. Isn't it great to know that there are always things that you can do to improve the way you live and deal with your condition?

In the remaining chapters of Part II, we'll discuss the different treatment options used for prostate cancer. The other aspects of an effective treatment program will be covered in subsequent parts of the book.

Chapter 5

SURGERY—REMOVING
THE PROSTATE GLAND

Not too many people cherish the thought of "going under the knife." But in the early stages of prostate cancer, when the cancer is confined to the prostate gland itself, many physicians consider surgery the treatment of choice. Usually, surgery is considered if you are no more than seventy years old or so and are in comparatively good health. Statistics suggest that approximately 10 percent of individuals with prostate cancer have surgery. Although not the most pleasant experience to consider, the benefits of surgery may make it worthwhile. So let's discuss surgery as one of the possible treatments for prostate cancer.

THE RADICAL PROSTATECTOMY

The surgical procedure used to treat early-stage prostate cancer is called *radical prostatectomy*. (Another type of surgery may be used in more advanced stages of prostate cancer. See Chapter 7 for details.) During Stages A2 and B, in which the cancer is contained within the prostate gland, this is the procedure preferred by many urologists.

The Surgery

In a radical prostatectomy, the entire prostate gland, the seminal vesicles, and the portion of the urethra near the bladder are removed. The neck of the bladder is then reconnected to the divided end of the urethra. The radical prostatectomy often takes from two to three hours.

How is the surgery performed? There are only two primary surgical approaches—the retropubic approach and the perineal approach.

In the *retropubic prostatectomy*, the surgical incision is made in the abdomen, and the surgeon approaches the gland from behind (retro) the pubic bone. In addition to the removal of the prostate gland, the seminal vesicles, and a portion of the urethra, nearby lymph nodes are also removed so that the surgeon can be sure that the cancer has not spread beyond the gland itself.

In the *perineal prostatectomy*, the gland is reached through the skin between the scrotum and the rectum. In this approach, because the surgeon cannot reach the lymph nodes, they are left intact.

Which is the better approach? In general, the choice of approach depends on a number of factors, the primary factory being the preference of the surgeon. However, the retropubic approach is considered to have two main advantages over the perineal approach. First, when using the retropubic technique, it's easier to save the nerves necessary for erection. Second, using this approach, there may be less danger of developing a loss of urinary control. So currently, the retropubic approach is used in most cases.

At the end of surgery, additional tissue surrounding the tumor is usually removed. This is done because commonly, cancerous tumors don't grow in self-contained, tight lumps. More often, the tumors have little root-like projections that branch off from the main body of the tumor. To make sure that all of these projections are removed, healthy tissue may also be removed.

The radical prostatectomy is not considered very painful surgery, thanks to the anesthesiologist, who administers anesthesia during the surgery itself, and the pain medication that you will be given for post-surgical discomfort. One of the new developments in pain control—which is discussed in more detail in Chapter 18—is the medication pump. If this is available in your hospital, you'll be able to administer your own medication just by pressing a button!

The Postsurgical Period

Following surgery, a catheter is used to drain the bladder and keep it at rest. The catheter is a rubber tube with a balloon on it. The tube extends through the penis to the bladder, where the balloon keeps it in place. This device minimizes postsurgical discomfort and helps promote healing before function is reestablished.

Most patients remain in the hospital for about seven days, but continue to use the catheter for two weeks after returning home. Yes, you might have a little discomfort in normal urination following catheter removal, but then again, you might not. Any symptoms, though, including urinary urgency, urinary frequency, and discomfort, can be controlled with appropriate medication.

All individuals experience incontinence—the inability to control urination—at least initially after surgery. Prepare yourself for this possibility. In fact, a degree of incontinence may be experienced for a month or two after the catheter is removed. Fortunately, though, the vast majority of people regain their ability to control urination, and have no further problems of this nature.

POSSIBLE SIDE EFFECTS OF SURGERY

Until recently, impotence was often a problem following prostate surgery, as surgery often resulted in the cutting or damaging of the nerves responsible for erection. In addition, in about 10 percent of all cases, permanent incontinence developed. However, more recent surgical procedures have been able to identify and separate the nerves that otherwise might have been cut, resulting in a significantly decreased likelihood of impotence and incontinence following surgery.

These nerve-sparing techniques, now more frequently employed in the retropubic surgical procedure, were first developed at Johns Hopkins University by Dr. Patrick Walsh. Dr. Walsh pinpointed the two bundles of nerves that are primarily responsible for controlling erection, and devised a surgical procedure that removes the prostate gland and capsule without damaging those nerves. And, in many cases, even if one of the bundles is inadvertently cut or damaged during surgery, sexual function can be maintained.

More and more urologists and surgeons are now becoming familiar with and using the Walsh procedure. It's estimated that these nerve-sparing surgical procedures for locally contained tumors can prevent impotence in 70 percent or more of all men who have prostate surgery. However, most surgeons try to prepare their patients for the possibility that they may become impotent as a result of the operation, and tell their patients that if impotence does not occur, they should consider it a plus. It's important to remember, though, that even when impotence does occur, the nerves that control orgasm may remain intact, and that, fortunately, there are devices and medications that can help a person regain sexual functioning. (More about this in Chapter 31.)

Certainly, other problems, as well, may occur as a result of prostate surgery. For example, although blood in the urine is never normal, it is inevitable following surgery. Remember that a little drop of blood in the urine can change the color of *all* the urine. This need not be cause for concern unless blood clots form and restrict the flow of urine. Of course, any problem with urination should be brought to your doctor's attention right away.

THINGS TO THINK ABOUT

If surgery is a possibility for you, there are a number of things that you should think about before making a decision:

☐ Get a second opinion. This is always important when deciding whether or not surgery is the best treatment for you. (See Chapter 29 for more information on getting a second opinion.)

☐ Ask your primary physician for recommendations regarding the best surgeon available for this procedure. Make sure that your surgeon is a specialist in prostate cancer.

☐ Because of the relative length of the operation, and because there is potential for considerable blood loss (there are a lot of veins near the pubic bone), you may want to store up two to four pints of your own blood prior to surgery, or have family members or friends with compatible blood types donate blood for you.

☐ Discuss what's involved in the operation, and what kind of rehabilitation will follow. What will you need to know before, during, and after the procedure?

☐ Speak to your doctor about using the watch-and-wait approach. Why? Most recent research studies show that, in the early stages, surgery may be no more effective than watchful waiting. Although each case is different, you may want to discuss this with your physician. Then consider both your doctor's opinion—especially if it's a strong one—and your own opinion before making a decision. If you and your doctor can't agree on the best course of action, you may want to explore your options further by consulting with other physicians. This is not to imply, though, that you should keep searching until you find a physician who endorses your view. If you continue to run into opposition, you may want to reconsider the facts.

Most important, feel free to ask questions. Remember that preparation for surgery will help give you the confidence and peace of mind you need to recuperate fully.

Chapter 6

RADIATION THERAPY

Many people with prostate cancer have radiation therapy at some time during their treatment. In fact, radiation therapy—also called radiotherapy, x-ray therapy, and irradiation—has been used to treat prostate cancer for many years. Only in the past quarter of a century, however, has the use of radiation been greatly improved both in effectiveness and in ease of application. Now, technology enables machines to deliver high-intensity rays in precise, carefully calculated doses to tumors deep within the body, with less damage to the organs and tissues that lie in between. These rays are used to slow or halt cancer cell growth, or to destroy all cancer cells. And, in many cases, radiation results in no change in sexual ability.

Let's learn a little bit more about how radiation therapy works, when it may be used as a treatment for prostate cancer, and how you can help control the side effects of this treatment.

WHAT DOES RADIATION THERAPY DO?

Radiation therapy uses high-level energy that affects any cells which are in the process of dividing. Since cancer cells divide more frequently than normal cells do, radiation is used in the hope that it will kill the cancer cells with minimal damage to the healthy tissues that surround them.

Radiation doesn't directly kill the cancer cells. Rather, it damages the DNA in the nucleus of the cancer cells, making it impossible for the cells to divide. And when cells don't divide, they die. So the goal is to hit cancer cells with radiation, damaging the DNA so the cells can no longer reproduce. The tumors then shrink rather than growing larger. In certain cases, in fact, radiation can completely destroy tumors. Even when destruction is not possible, the tumor shrinkage resulting from radiation can sometimes make the tumor more amenable to surgery, or can at least prolong life.

HOW IS RADIATION USED TO TREAT PROSTATE CANCER?

There are three ways in which radiation can be used to treat prostate cancer. First, when prostate cancer is localized, radiation can be used as a curative procedure by aiming the rays at the gland itself and at the lymph nodes in the immediate area. In this case, the ten-year cure rate using radiation is considered to be approximately the same as that for surgery. Of course, radiation is usually not nearly as physically or emotionally distressing as surgery, and there are fewer complications, as well.

Second, radiation therapy may be used on individuals whose cancer has spread a little beyond the prostate. When this is the case, the radiation is directed not only toward the prostate, but toward the whole pelvic area, including the nearby lymph nodes.

Finally, radiation can be used to alleviate pain. For instance, prostate cancer that has metastasized to the bone can be quite painful, and radiation therapy can often both reduce the pain and lessen the risk of cancer-related fractures. Radiation can also decrease the size of tumors that cause pain by pressing on nerve endings.

THE TWO TYPES OF RADIATION THERAPY

There are two ways in which prostate cancer can be treated with radiation. The radiation can be delivered externally, with machines that emit rays in precise doses, or internally, through the use of implants.

External Radiation Treatment

External radiation, a technique commonly used in the treatment of cancer, involves the beaming of rays from an external source to an exposed part of the body. The radiation is directed at the specific area pinpointed by the radiation oncologist in collaboration with the urologist. Usually, either a radiation oncologist or a radiation therapist uses a special type of indelible ink to mark the part of the body where the radiation is to be focused. There is normally no sensation during treatment.

Most often, external radiation treatments are performed on an outpatient basis, and are administered each weekday for six to seven weeks. Treatment is extended over a period of time so that the doses of radiation can remain small, minimizing any possible side effects to the rectum or bladder. Each individual treatment usually lasts for only about one to five minutes. Once the treatment is over, no residual radioactivity remains in the body. It should be noted that because the doses of radiation are so carefully calculated, there is no need to monitor the patient for radiation exposure.

Radiation Implants

Internal radiation—also called interstitial radiation—a technique newer than external radiation, is also an established treatment for many cancers, including prostate cancer. Implantation involves the placing of a seed of radioactive material in a part of the body, a body cavity, or a tissue. In the treatment of prostate cancer, this is done using a long needle that is inserted through the perineum—the area between the scrotum and the rectum. The radioactive material used in these seeds is most often iodine or palladium, a metal similar to platinum.

The advantage of placing implants directly in the prostate is that higher doses of radiation can then be directly applied to the tumor, with minimal damage—called "scatter"—to adjacent tissues and organs. Because of the highly localized effect of this treatment, implants are used only when the cancer is in its earliest stages. The implants are not used once the cancer has spread to the bones or lymph nodes.

Radioactive implants are left permanently inside the prostate. These implants do not continue to function indefinitely, though, but stop emitting radiation within a short period of time, usually a few months. Once in place, the implants do not cause any discomfort.

One of the reasons that internal radiation is used less frequently than external radiation is that it requires a surgical procedure. However, this surgery, which is often guided by ultrasound imaging, is a relatively simple procedure, and can sometimes be performed on an outpatient basis. Internal radiation, like external radiation, need not be monitored, as the dose of radiation is carefully calculated before the seeds are implanted.

POSSIBLE SIDE EFFECTS OF RADIATION THERAPY

Radiation usually has few side effects and complications, but side effects do occur. Most of these side effects are the result of external radiation, as this type of treatment can damage the healthy cells around the prostate. Fewer side effects are experienced when radiation implants are used.

Most types of side effects can be acute or chronic. Acute reactions are those that usually occur soon after radiation has begun, and disappear within a few weeks or months, although they may last longer. Chronic reactions usually develop more slowly and last for a longer period of time—in some cases, months or years. The nature of the side effects that each individual experiences depends on the type of radiation used and the focus of the radiation.

One common side effect of both internal and external radiation is fatigue. Normally, though, this fatigue is not so bad that it prevents you from working or from continuing your normal activities.

Radiation may also cause skin problems—usually when external rays penetrate the skin to reach the cancerous cells below. Often, the irradiated area of the body looks sunburned—a problem that is mild, but chronic in nature. A more severe reaction might be a decrease in healing ability or a burning sensation of the skin. Or a rash may appear in the irradiated area.

Another possible side effect of both internal and external radiation therapy is a further narrowing of the urethra, which can cause urinary difficulties. There may also be rectal inflammation, which can occasionally cause bleeding or diarrhea. Bladder inflammation—cystitis, sometimes called radiation cystitis—may also occur, leading to urination problems, such as feelings of urinary urgency and frequency, and blood in the urine.

Like cancer cells, the cells that line the walls of the intestines normally divide quickly. As a result, both internal and external radiation can damage these cells, causing diarrhea and rectal irritation.

Chronic impotence, too, is a fairly frequent side effect of radiation therapy for prostate cancer, and most commonly results from external treatments. Some studies suggest that 20 percent or more of the men who undergo this treatment may experience impotence. There are reported cases in which erectile dysfunctions were not immediately present, but appeared one or two years after the radiation treatment. Other studies, however, suggest that impotence is not a common result of radiation therapy.

Men who have external radiation treatments for prostate cancer may lose their pubic hair. One of the reasons for this is that hair follicle cells—like cancer cells, and also like the cells that line the intestines—divide much more quickly and frequently than most other cells do. Because of this, radiation-induced DNA damage affects these cells in much the same way it affects the cancer cells. And when hair cells are not able to reproduce because of DNA damage, hair falls out.

COPING WITH THE SIDE EFFECTS OF RADIATION THERAPY

Physicians can prescribe medication to control many of the side effects just discussed. But are there any things you can do to help? Of course there are!

Skin that has been exposed to radiation—called irradiated skin—is very sensitive. The side effects of radiation tend to be worse when the tissue that is irradiated is already diseased or infected. But even when the skin is healthy, care must be taken to protect it from tight clothing, heat, sun, and other things that could cause irritation. For instance, during radiation therapy, it is important to avoid using strong or perfumed soaps around the affected area. Also to be avoided are heat lamps, hot water bottles, and colognes. And if skin reactions do occur—often in the form of red, itchy, flaky skin—you might try soothing the area with a very light baby oil or another unscented moisturizer. You might also try applying corn starch as a powder. Of course, you should contact your doctor as soon as problems appear. If necessary, he may prescribe hydrocortisone cream or another type of treatment.

Good nutrition is also essential during radiation therapy. It is vital to take in appropriate amounts of healthy foods and liquids in order to strengthen the immune system, maintain your weight, and prevent digestive problems. Also, the right nutrients will help your body rebuild any tissues damaged by radiation. (See Chapter 21 for more information on diet, and Chapter 20 for more information on the control of side effects.)

Finally, remember that everyone who undergoes treatment for prostate cancer is unique. You may have a number of these symptoms—or you may feel quite well throughout your radiation treatments. If problems do occur, though, be sure to speak to your doctor, who should be able to answer all your questions and to help you cope with any side effects.

Chapter 7

HORMONE THERAPY

Tumors that have spread, or metastasized, beyond the prostate gland to the lymph nodes, bone, and, possibly, various organs, are not considered curable. In many cases of metastasis, though, hormone therapy—also called hormone manipulation—has been successfully used to suppress and control symptoms and minimize further spread.

Hormone therapy techniques may sound drastic and almost always affect sexual function, and hormone therapy cannot *cure* cancer. However, this therapy can lead to remission, and can bring about prompt relief from pain—relief that can last for several years!

THE TWO TYPES OF HORMONE THERAPY

As discussed earlier in the book, it is known that the growth of prostate cancer is dependent on the male hormone testosterone. So, logically, if testosterone is eliminated, prostate cancer may be more controllable. In fact, it has been found that regardless of how far the prostate cancer has spread—to the lymph glands, bones, lungs, or other parts of the body— by eliminating the source of growth stimulation, namely the male hormone testosterone, malignant cells can be destroyed. In some cases, cancer diagnosed beyond the range acceptable for prostate-gland removal has been reduced through hormone therapy to the point at which treatment by that type of surgery is possible. This treatment may even lead to remission.

There are two main ways in which testosterone can be eliminated. In the first approach, the source of the testosterone is removed. Many males may cringe at this idea, because we're talking about removing the testicles (castration). As unpleasant at this may sound, though, this relatively painless procedure is considered to be the most direct way of depriving the cancer of its main source of growth stimulation.

The other method of depriving prostate cancer tumors of their testosterone supply is to chemically remove the hormone by administering a substance that suppresses testosterone production.

So hormonal manipulation involves removing the testicles or administering antihormonal agents. Or these methods may be used in combination. Let's discuss these two approaches in more detail.

Removal of the Testicles (Orchiectomy)

Bilateral orchiectomy—also called orchidectomy—is the removal of both testicles, and is used to reduce or eliminate the source of testosterone, the male hormone that stimulates prostate cancer growth. For many surgeons, orchiectomy is the treatment of choice whenever it is recognized that prostate cancer has metastasized. Other surgeons do not recommend orchiectomy until the metastasis is widespread. Orchiectomy is usually not recommended when the cancer is contained totally within the prostate gland.

Orchiectomy is a relatively simple, painless procedure. It is performed under either a local or general anesthetic, and usually requires only an overnight hospital stay followed by a three- to four-day period of recuperation.

After the testicles are removed, the scrotal bag remains intact, although empty. If the patient is uncomfortable with an empty scrotal sack, it can be filled with a synthetic substance so that the outward appearance is the same that it was prior to surgery.

Hormone Suppression

Many men prefer not to undergo the orchiectomy. Because the key to hormone therapy is elimination of the male hormone testosterone, the other primary technique used in hormone therapy involves the chemical suppression of testosterone production. In many individuals, this approach has been just as successful as testicle removal. In others, a combination of these two approaches has been the most successful.

Years ago, female hormones were used to counteract the male hormones. Diethylstilbestrol (DES), a synthetic form of estrogen, was one medication prescribed for this purpose. But large doses of the drug were necessary to suppress testosterone production. Worse, the men who used the medication would develop many of the same side effects developed by women who take estrogen, including water retention and thrombophlebitis (inflammation of a vein often accompanied by blood clot formation). So the best means of reducing or eliminating testosterone was still orchiectomy.

Fortunately, in the past few years, other methods of testosterone suppression have been developed, including the drug Lupron (leuprolide acetate). Lupron is called an LH-RH agonist. This means that instead of trying to block the testosterone—or "antagonize" it—the drug causes the cells in the testicles to produce so much testosterone that they become exhausted and shut down production.

Of course, there are problems associated with Lupron's initial effect of increasing testosterone production. For instance, when a person has bone pain due to metastasis, the administration of Lupron causes more testosterone production and, as a result, increased tumor growth and increased pain. For this reason, before administering Lupron, doctors may administer Eulixin (flutamide), which interferes with the binding of male hormones to prostate cancer cells. After a week to ten days on Eulixin, the monthly injections of Lupron are begun—with no increase in testosterone production.

Is Eulixin used after Lupron injections begin? Sometimes, after a period of time, an increased level of prostate-specific antigen indicates that another gland—the adrenal gland—is producing testosterone. When this is determined, Eulixin is used to stop the adrenal gland's production of the hormone.

Unfortunately, both Lupron and Eulixin are quite expensive, and Eulixin has the added problem of causing diarrhea and gastric upsets. Because of these drawbacks, as well as the effort involved in getting monthly injections of Lupron, many men eventually opt for bilateral orchiectomy.

POSSIBLE SIDE EFFECTS OF HORMONE THERAPY

Men need not be concerned that either type of hormone therapy will result in a high voice and loss of facial hair. These problems arise only when a man loses his testicles before puberty. If a man has had full male hormones throughout his life, there should not be any noticeable voice, appearance, or personality changes following bilateral orchiectomy or hormone suppression.

As already mentioned, hormone suppression may lead to gastric upset. Another unpleasant side effect—one that can result from either type of hormone therapy—is hot flashes. This side effect, although uncomfortable, is usually not so serious that doctors discontinue therapy. Some men, however, experience these flashes two or three times a day, and sometimes more frequently, much the way women do when going through menopause.

More upsetting to most men is that, eventually, both orchiectomy and hormone suppression result in impotence. While some men experience sexual desire for up to a year after surgery, erectile capabilities are absent due to the elimination of testosterone.

COPING WITH THE SIDE EFFECTS OF HORMONE THERAPY

Fortunately, there is help available for men coping with the side effects of hormone therapy. When gastric upset results from hormone suppression, medication may be able to lessen this problem. The chosen medication will, of course, depend on the nature of the upset.

When hot flashes cause great discomfort, the drug Provera (medroxyprogesterone acetate)—a derivative of the female hormone progesterone—is one of the medications that may provide help. Most men, however, prefer to ride out these episodes without medication. In a number of cases, the frequency of hot flashes has tapered off with time.

Although intercourse is not the only means of deriving sexual pleasure, many men, quite understandably, seek to regain sexual function after hormone therapy. For these men, a number of effective medications and devices may prove helpful. See Chapter 31 for detailed information on sex and prostate cancer.

Hormone therapy can be an effective means of shrinking prostate cancer, halting its growth, and relieving pain and other symptoms. If your doctor has recommended hormone therapy, be sure to discuss the available options and to have all of your questions answered. Once you fully understand each of the different elements of your treatment program, you'll be better able to cope with prostate cancer.

Chapter 8

ALTERNATIVE TREATMENTS

So far, this book has provided you with a great deal of information on the three conventional prostate cancer treatments most often used in our country—namely, surgery, radiation, and hormone therapy. Much research continues to explore better ways of using these accepted methods of treatment.

However, a growing number of people are now also interested in learning about alternative treatments—also called nontoxic therapies, complementary treatments, nonconventional therapies, and, by critics, unorthodox approaches. Why? Many people with cancer want to find the best possible ways of treating their disease. They may want to use alternative therapies as a means of strengthening their bodies and controlling side effects while undergoing conventional treatment. Or they may prefer the gentler, noninvasive approach of alternative therapies.

Let's learn more about alternative therapies—about how they aim to treat cancer, about the many different alternative therapies available, and about how you can choose an alternative therapy that may help you cope better with prostate cancer.

SIMILARITIES OF ALTERNATIVE TREATMENTS

Despite the fact that there are a number of different types of alternative treatments, they do have common "themes." Perhaps the best way to begin a discussion of alternative treatments is to look at the common philosophies behind many of these different treatments.

Many of the alternative therapies are based on the belief that a truly healthy body is much less vulnerable to cancer. They emphasize that cancer develops because of a problem with the immune system or an imbalance in the body, either or both of which permit the development of the cancer. All alternative methods are designed to create (or re-create) the healthiest possible body—to reduce or eliminate the immune system problem or imbalance that allowed the cancer to develop in the first place. Some alternative practitioners state that the body should first be detoxified through a cleansing process. The hope, of course, is that this increasingly healthy state will activate the body's healing process so that it is able to eliminate the cancer.

Alternative treatments are basically nontoxic. This contrasts with radiation or chemotherapy, which may destroy normal cells, causing side effects and weakening the body. Instead, alternative treatments aim at strengthening the body.

Alternative treatments usually use a wholistic approach—that is, their goal is to treat the whole body, rather than just the area seemingly affected by the cancer. Most are based on the idea that although the cancer may be found in one particular area, the entire system is involved. Therefore, the body must be treated as a whole. Many also aim to treat the body on a number of different levels, including physical, mental, spiritual, and emotional levels.

CATEGORIES OF ALTERNATIVE TREATMENTS

There are a number of different categories of alternative treatments, including biologic and pharmacologic therapies, immune therapies, herbal therapies, metabolic therapies, mind-body therapies, and nutritional therapies. As you read the following discussions and learn which specific treatments and programs may be used in each category, keep in mind that there is a certain amount of overlap between the categories regarding approaches and techniques. For instance, an immune therapy may use diet as part of its program, and a nutritional therapy may seek to strengthen the immune system. However, these categories do serve to highlight the central focus of each treatment or regimen.

Biologic and Pharmacologic Therapies

These therapies use biologic substances or nontoxic pharmacologic agents—nontoxic medications usually derived from a biological source, such as plants or human cells. Each of these therapies works in a different way. For instance, antineoplaston therapy, which uses amino-acid derivatives, is said to inhibit the growth of cancer cells; and hydrazine sulfate, a nontoxic off-the-shelf chemical, is said to have antitumor action and to stimulate appetite and weight gain. Another treatment in this category is Revici therapy, which aims at correcting an underlying imbalance in the body. Finally, shark cartilage—a natural food substance—is a promising new therapy that is now the focus of much research. Shark cartilage is thought to work by blocking angiogenesis, the creation of new capillary blood vessels required for tumor growth, and thus starving the tumor of needed nourishment.

Immune Therapies

Immune therapies are based on the belief that cancer develops because of a breakdown of the immune system. The aim of these therapies is to bolster those parts of the immune system that combat and destroy cancer cells. Examples of the treatments in this category include Dr. Lawrence Burton's Immuno-Augmentative Therapy (IAT), which uses four blood proteins found to restore normal immune function; the therapy of Dr. Virginia Livingston, which uses vaccines, diet, nutritional supplements, and gamma globulin; and Dr. Josef Issels' whole-body therapy, which uses vaccines, diet, and fever therapy.

Herbal Therapies

In these therapies, probably the oldest form of treatment in the world is used to strengthen the body's ability to eliminate cancer cells. Hoxsey therapy employs internal and external herbal preparations, along with diet, vitamin and mineral supplements, and psychological counseling to strengthen the body and fight the cancer. Substances used in various other herbal therapies include essiac, an herbal tea; mistletoe extract; pau d'arco tea; and chaparral tea.

Metabolic Therapies

These therapies are based on the idea that many factors cause the occurrence of cancer, and that a multifaceted healing approach is required to eliminate the disorder. The therapies use detoxification, including colon cleansing, to flush out toxins that interfere with proper metabolism; anticancer diets based on whole foods; and vitamins, minerals, and enzymes, which further cleanse the body, repair damaged tissues, and stimulate immune function. Examples of metabolic therapies include Dr. Max Gerson's therapy, which bases its program on organically grown fresh fruits and vegetables, as well as supplements; Dr. William Kelley's nutritional-metabolic therapy, which involves therapeutic nutrition, anticancer supplements, and vigorous detoxification; and Dr. Hans Nieper's therapy, a complex metabolic-nutritional program that employs diet, supplements, laetrile, drugs, and other components.

Mind-Body Therapies

These treatments focus on the role that emotions, behavior, and faith play in the recovery from illness. In the case of some therapies, counseling, hypnosis, biofeedback, or other techniques are used to promote greater emotional and spiritual well-being. In other therapies, the aim is to use mind-body techniques to actually change the course of the illness, possibly bringing the person into remission. Dr. O. Carl Simonton and Stephanie Matthews-Simonton, for instance, developed a visualization technique designed to help patients increase the effectiveness of their immune systems. The Simontons' programs include psychotherapy, a discussion of diet and exercise, and other components.

Nutritional Therapies

Therapies that focus on nutrition are perhaps the most popular alternative approach, especially now that research has clearly indicated a link between diet and health. Studies have shown, for instance, that high-fat diets increase the risk of cancer, while low-fat diets that are rich in fiber, fresh fruits and vegetables, and whole grains, actually help our bodies fight cancer. Three of the therapies that fall into this category are wheatgrass therapy, a diet based on wheatgrass and other "live" (uncooked) foods; the macrobiotic diet, a traditional Japanese diet high in whole grains and vegetables; and the Moerman regimen, a meatless high-fiber diet used with eight supplements. (See Chapter 21 for more information on diet.)

Keep in mind that the above discussion by no means mentions all of the categories of alternative treatments, nor does it include all of the individual therapies. For instance, other therapies you may hear about are bioelectric therapy, homeopathy, oxygen therapy, hyperthermia, chelation, and live-cell therapy. However, this discussion should make you aware of the many types of treatments that are available.

CHOOSING A TREATMENT THAT'S RIGHT FOR YOU

Ironically, in choosing an alternative treatment that's right for you, your first step should be to learn about conventional treatments. Why? It's important to fully understand what the available conventional treatments are, why your doctor recommends them, and what both the benefits and the side effects may be. Even if you feel that you would prefer an alternative treatment, you owe it to yourself to find out what *all* your options are.

You can learn about both conventional and alternative therapies from a number of sources. By visiting libraries and bookstores and contacting health organizations that focus on cancer, you should be able to find a number of comprehensive, up-to-date books that provide additional information both about your cancer and about the available treatments. For example, Richard Walters' *Options: The Alternative Cancer Therapy Book* can help you to evaluate and compare a number of alternative cancer therapies.

In learning about conventional treatments, you'll probably find your doctor to be a valuable resource. While you're talking to your physician, though, don't hesitate to ask him about alternative treatments too. He or she may have had patients who tried various alternative therapies, or may know of professionals with some experience with unorthodox treatments. Of course, if you're very interested in alternative therapies and your doctor seems skeptical—even discouraging—you may wish to look for a doctor who is more sympathetic to your point of view. Keep in mind, though, that you may *never* find a doctor willing to support you in your use of alternative therapies. Therefore, if you do choose to use one or more nonconventional therapies, you will have to assume greater responsibility for your own well-being than is usually required under the care of a conventional practitioner. The responsibility will be yours to perform your own research and participate actively in your own recovery.

If the doctors you contact aren't able to help you evaluate the alternative therapies you're interested in, contact educational organizations and patient-referral services that provide information on these treatments. *Options*, mentioned above, provides a list of these groups. John Fink's *Third Opinion: An International Directory to Alternative Therapy Centers for the Treatment and Prevention of Cancer and Other Degenerative Diseases* is another good source of information on alternative therapies. (See the reading list on page 277 for further titles.)

When looking into a particular therapy, try to get information from other people who have prostate cancer. Some information organizations, and some alternative clinics, as well, have lists of recovered patients whom you can call or write to. Don't hesitate to contact these people and see what they specifically did that helped them.

When screening alternative practitioners and clinics, ask what their success has been in treating prostate cancer. How many cases of prostate cancer do they see every year? Keep in mind that a therapy that's effective against one type of cancer isn't necessarily effective against yours. Ask to see supportive studies, documented cases, and patients' testimonials. View all information with a healthy dose of skepticism, and pin the practitioners down as much as possible about whether you can expect long-term improvement, short-term improvement, long-term survival, or reduced pain. Also ask if the therapy is being used instead of, or in addition to, conventional treatment. More and more widely respected medical practitioners are now combining the best aspects of conventional medicine with supportive alternative treatments.

Finally, consider whether a therapy fits in with your lifestyle, personality, and belief system. Some therapies, for instance, may require a degree of commitment that you are not willing or able to make. Some may require more time than you have—especially if you work full-time—or too much travel. And some may simply be too expensive.

AN ALTERNATIVE CONCLUSION

In learning to cope with prostate cancer, your choice of treatment will be one of the most important decisions you'll make. To make the best possible decision, you'll want to learn as much as you can about all available treatments, both conventional and alternative, and to consider the facts carefully.

Once you choose a treatment, do your best to follow through and to give the program a fair trial. Be alert to the progress being made, and stay open to trying something new if the treatment you're using either isn't working or is working against you.

PART III

YOUR EMOTIONS

Chapter 9

COPING WITH YOUR EMOTIONS— AN INTRODUCTION

How do you feel about having prostate cancer? What a question! The diagnosis of prostate cancer can have a tremendous emotional impact on you, your family, your friends—on everyone around you.

Each person's emotional responses to prostate cancer are different. Even your own reactions to the condition will vary from time to time. The more severe your reactions are, the more they will interfere with your ability to cope. Your emotions can ride a roller coaster. In other words, you may feel relatively okay at some times, and very down at others. As a matter of fact, emotional ups and downs are very common. But one of the most important ingredients in being able to cope with prostate cancer is the ability to remain in control of your emotions.

Your emotional reactions to prostate cancer may start even before treatment has begun. Of course, your reaction will partly depend on how suddenly you found out you had it. For example, if, without any warning symptoms, you were suddenly diagnosed with prostate cancer, you might not adjust as well as you would if you had been experiencing symptoms for a while, and had suspected that a problem existed.

THE FACTORS SHAPING YOUR EMOTIONAL REACTIONS

A number of factors may play a role in determining how you react to prostate cancer. Keep in mind, though, that because there are so many factors, no one can predict how any person will react at any given time. How did you handle problems before your condition was diagnosed? What was your general coping style? Were you calm or nervous? Were you persistent or did you give up easily? The way you've handled life's problems in general will suggest how well you can cope with prostate cancer and its treatment, and which areas you'll want to improve.

Your age will also have a bearing on how you respond emotionally. And your general physical health prior to the onset of prostate cancer will also play a role in determining your coping ability. What about your relationships? In many cases, your emotional reactions may reflect the responses of significant others in your life. For example, if family members or friends are anxious about your medical condition, this may very well affect the way you feel.

WHAT EMOTIONAL PROBLEMS?

Have you been experiencing intense anger because you have to go through all this? Are you angry that your life will change because of prostate cancer? Are you afraid of cancer in general? Are you afraid of the treatment you may need? Are you afraid of not being able to cope? Do you become depressed when you compare your present life with the way things were? Virtually everyone who is diagnosed with cancer is anxious, frightened, and depressed. Feeling this way doesn't mean that you are weak. Rather, it means that you are normal! Because of the importance of coping with these emotions, a separate chapter has been devoted to each of them. But other than these specific emotional responses, what else might you experience?

You may feel disoriented—as if the things around you are unreal. One of the most frightening feelings is that you're not yourself, especially if you don't know why you're feeling this way. It can be reassuring to understand that this happens to many people from time to time. And it can go away.

How about mood swings? Do you ever experience these? Many individuals with prostate cancer do. But if you stop to think about it, everyone experiences mood swings from time to time, whether they have prostate cancer or not! It is possible that certain treatments or medications may even increase the range or frequency of these mood swings. Let your physician know what's going on so that appropriate changes can be made.

THREE TIMES OF CRISIS

In general, there are three main emotional crises that occur when people have cancer. The first crisis occurs when the person is initially diagnosed. The second occurs when he has to begin cancer treatment. And the third occurs when he finds out that he's going to die—but hopefully, you'll never encounter this one!

There are some experts who feel that there is even a fourth crisis—one that occurs when the individual finds out that treatment has been successful and that he's going to live! Why is this a crisis? Although this may seem to be the desired outcome, the individual now has to worry about recurrences and future health problems.

THE PROCESS OF ADJUSTING

You—as well as your family—will probably experience a number of major emotional reactions as part of the adjustment process. Shock and disbelief, anger, denial, depression, uncertainty, and fear are all normal responses when faced with a diagnosis of prostate cancer. Later in this part of the book, there are complete chapters devoted to anger, depression, and fear. But what about the others? Let's take a look at the remaining emotions, and also at a number of other feelings you may experience during your adjustment process and beyond.

Shock and Disbelief

Being diagnosed with prostate cancer can certainly be shocking. And as the intensity of the shock wears off, it is quickly replaced by feelings of disbelief. It's hard to believe that you've got cancer. This disbelief, though, is actually a calmer sensation than initial shock and subsequent emotions. It gives you a chance to adjust to what you have heard—to get used to it in your own way, at your own speed.

Give yourself a chance to get used to the diagnosis of cancer. Don't feel that you have to absorb it—or, more important, accept it—all at once. This takes time.

Denial

It can be very difficult for someone to accept the fact that he has cancer. So instead of acceptance, he may experience denial. And denial can lead to delays in treatment.

Believe it or not, there are times when denial can be a positive technique. How? It can be helpful by keeping you from dwelling on problems that aren't improved by dwelling! In other words, if there's nothing you can do to make a situation better, why keep thinking about it? Remember that denial does distort reality, but that there may be times when distortion is necessary. So denial can be helpful early on, following diagnosis, as you get used to dealing with that diagnosis. It may enable you to go about normal routines while you're getting used to these unpleasant circumstances. It may help you maintain hope, which is necessary in continuing to do the things you have to do. But the appropriateness of denial can turn to inappropriateness if it keeps you from doing what you have to do in order to help yourself.

Family members deny also. But when family members allow denial to continue, they may be contributing to, or enabling, a person's inappropriate way of dealing with the problem.

Uncertainty

There is always uncertainty in our lives. But rarely does this uncertainty become as obvious as it does when you've been diagnosed with cancer. Now you're faced with uncertainties from this point on—uncertainty regarding treatment, outcome, symptoms, and so on.

Uncertainty exists regardless of treatment outcome. Even if there is success in treatment, there still can be uncertainty as to future outcome, future recurrences, and future problems. Always have hope. But be realistic. Don't deceive yourself. Remember that you are able to move in only one direction at a time. Instead of focusing on the uncertainty in your life, focus on the certainty. Do the things you normally do. Don't play the role of a sick person. Get on with the act of living.

Focus on the quality rather than the quantity of your life. Make the most of each day, rather than figuring out how many days you have to make the most of. Focus on what you have, not on what you've lost.

Work to change your attitude. Instead of saying, "Cancer is something you die from," try to say, "Cancer is something you learn to live with."

Damaged Self-Esteem

One of the most important characteristics that each of us has is our self-esteem. The way you feel about yourself is very important and helps you get through the day. Unfortunately, a diagnosis of cancer can certainly have a damaging effect on your self-esteem.

Have you liked yourself less since your diagnosis? Previous feelings of confidence can be quickly shattered, and this can have a very unpleasant effect. You may not feel or behave like yourself. You'll want to deal with this right away in order to return to effective, efficient functioning.

One problem that can affect your self-esteem is the feeling that you're no longer independent and that you've lost some control over your life. Although the degree to which independence is lost varies from person to person, everybody experiences a little less independence and a little less control because of cancer. Medical visits, treatments, waiting to hear from others about "the next step"—all these things make you more dependent on the medical system. And this may continue for the rest of your life. Your self-esteem may suffer if you feel more dependent on others at home or in the hospital, where virtually every aspect of your life is controlled by others.

What can you do about this? Instead of being upset by the things you can't do or the ways in which you are dependent on others, focus on the things you still can do! Take control over as much of your life as possible. Get involved in support programs and rehabilitation programs, and speak to others to find out how they handle these very important areas. If necessary, speak to professionals to get additional tips.

Changing Body Image

Changes in body image may occur because of surgery, radiation treatments, or hormone therapy. In fact, just knowing you have cancer can change the way you feel about your body. This can have a very profound effect on your self-esteem.

Body changes may include skin discoloration, scars, hair loss, weight loss, and so on. Cancer treatment that focuses on the male reproductive organs may be very upsetting in itself. It may make you think—inappropriately!—that you're not really a man.

What can you do to improve your body image? Consider the changes that have affected you the most, and speak to experts to learn about things that you can do to eliminate or lessen any problems. For instance, a different style of clothing may refocus the attention of others; makeup—yes, men can and do wear makeup—can camouflage scars and other skin problems; and dietary programs can stabilize weight. Remember that because of the location of the prostate cancer, many body changes may not be noticeable to others—except at very intimate times, when passion may reduce their importance, anyway. So the most significant step you can take may be to work on your attitude. Remind yourself of who you are, and who you've always been. Feel good about the things that are truly important, and minimize the rest.

Self-Blame

You may have read or heard that some people believe that you "set yourself up" for cancer. This may make you feel that if you've got cancer, you brought it on yourself! Another very unfortunate emotional reaction to cancer is the thought that you're being punished for something you did—that the disease is the result of some wrongdoing. What's the point of thinking this way? Does it really help you? It isn't true, so why let these thoughts overwhelm you?

There's no question that there is a connection between mind and body. There's no question that the way you feel can contribute to the way your health thrives or suffers. But rather than spending valuable energy blaming yourself for ways in which you may have let your body down, doesn't it make more sense to focus on ways in which you can build your body up, correct any problems that you can work on correcting, and move on? One of the best ways you can do this is to work on improving the way you deal with your emotions. Therefore, you'll want to recognize and let go of any self-blame. Not only do you want to be compassionate towards others, but you want to be compassionate towards yourself! Try to focus on what you can do to improve yourself, both physically and emotionally. Prepare yourself for as long and happy a life as possible.

Negative Thoughts

It is as important to push away negative thoughts as it is to eliminate self-blame. The less room there is in your mental attitude for negativity, the more room there will be for positive feelings. This will provide you with an important foundation in your efforts to get better.

Everyone has negative thoughts—thoughts that lead to the growth and intensity of negative emotions. However, there is no law that says that you have to allow these thoughts to continue to affect you. There is no law that says that you must allow them to remain in your head and overwhelm you. Keep challenging these thoughts. Keep working to turn them around and make them more rational, realistic, and positive. In this way, you'll continue to have hope, and continue to focus on the positive feelings that are such an essential part of successfully living with cancer.

It is a waste of valuable energy to be angry, guilty, self-blaming, or self-critical. It's now time to harness the energy that goes into these negative emotions and turn them into positive energy that can strengthen you.

MANAGING EMOTIONAL REACTIONS

Because your emotions play such an important role in your life with prostate cancer, you'll certainly want to do the best possible job you can of controlling them. How? Let's discuss some of the more important ways in which you can manage your emotions.

Gather Information

Always stay up-to-date on the latest information on your cancer and its treatment, and on any other information that may be helpful to you. Learn as much as you can. More people are afraid of what they don't know than what they do know. You want to be as educated as possible. In that way, you will best be able to help yourself, both in dealing with others—family, friends, and professionals—and in controlling your own emotional state.

Join a Support Group

Self-help or support groups can be incredibly helpful, and are one of the best sources of support for people who have cancer. Groups provide a forum for the exchange of feelings and ideas. Perhaps most important, these groups will show you that you're not alone. And it is much easier to live with a difficult problem when you know that you're not alone. It's helpful to meet new people—people other than family and friends— who know what you're going through because they've gone through it themselves.

All of the people in support groups have a common goal: to learn how to live as best as they can, to do as much as they possibly can. You'll see how others handle problems, some of which may be the same as, or at least similar to, your own. Learning how other people cope can be a tremendous source of support, especially if you really want to cope better but you're not always sure how to do it.

There are many groups that are run by professional leaders or facilitators that can be helpful to those who have prostate cancer. These groups are great places to share your feelings and gain valuable information and strategies in a constructive, therapeutically beneficial way, because of the expertise of the professional leading the group. Remember that groups are not designed to give false hope. They are designed to enable you to express and share real feelings, and to offer real strategies and hope for individuals living in similar circumstances.

Support groups can also be wonderful for your family, giving spouses, children, parents, and others the chance to get some support of their own. And since one of the best ways to be in control of your emotions is to have a supportive family behind you, you should most certainly encourage the participation of your family members.

Do you ever feel shunned or ignored by others—or do you fear feeling this way? Are your social relationships dwindling? Groups can give you a feeling of belonging.

In groups, any topics you'd like to talk about can be discussed. You may begin to share feelings more openly when you hear others talking about subjects you were previously reluctant to bring up yourself. As a result, a feeling of closeness—almost a family feeling—will develop.

Many times, members of groups dealing with chronic medical conditions discuss feelings of hostility towards the medical profession. A person alone with these feelings may have a hard time communicating with and trusting his physicians. In a group, hopefully, the feelings experienced can be straightened out so that a more positive, constructive relationship can be formed with medical professionals. (See Chapter 29 for more information on coping with physicians.)

Some people are afraid of what they're going to see if they go to a group meeting. They fear that they'll see people who are much sicker than they are, and that this will frighten them, negating any positive benefits. If this is one of your concerns, before attending a meeting, make sure to speak to whomever runs the group to learn about the group's composition.

Don't feel that you *have* to be in a group. If you're really uncomfortable with the idea, or you really don't think it's necessary because you're involved in other support activities, that's okay. Just make sure that you're honest with yourself. And don't feel that you *have* to share your emotional reactions with others. It's not necessary to talk them out, even though this can be helpful. But do realize that these emotions need to be recognized and worked through. That's the only way to make progress.

There are many different types of support groups. The list of resource groups on page 279 may help you locate some of them. The most well-known groups that deal with prostate cancer are those set up by the American Cancer Society, Cancer Care, and other organizations of this type. Other support groups may be found in hospice organizations, religious organizations, libraries, councils on aging, and so on.

The American Cancer Society is well known for the services it offers to individuals and family members living with cancer. One of the society's programs is called "I Can Cope." This is offered throughout the country, and provides information about different types of cancers, different therapies and treatments, nutrition, medication, side effects, and other topics that may be of interest to those with cancer and to their family members.

The American Cancer Society also operates a short-term "visitor program." Called "CanSurmount," this program helps patients and family members deal with many different types of cancer. Counseling is usually offered on a one-to-one basis.

Get the Best Medical Care Possible

Make sure you're getting the best possible medical care. If you haven't already done so, you'll want to establish a good working relationship with a physician. This involves seeing a doctor who not only has expertise in treating prostate cancer and has kept informed of the most up-to-date research, but is also understanding, available, and sympathetic to your emotional needs. You'll want to be sure that your physician monitors your condition so that any problems that may arise can be successfully treated. And if you're currently involved in treatment, you'll want your physician to monitor this, too, so that the therapy proceeds the way it's supposed to, and any side effects are minimized. (See Chapter 29 for tips on creating a good relationship with your physician.)

Learn About Medications That Can Help You Cope

There are times when emotions may get too intense. In some of these cases, you may want to consider medications that can help you cope. A number of medications can be effective in dealing with depression, anxiety, anger, and many other emotional manifestations of cancer. Antianxiety medication can be helpful, as can mood elevators and antidepressants. (More about this in Chapter 18.) Remember that your doctor is the one who is in charge of medication. Don't "play with fire." On the other hand, if a prescribed medication has unpleasant or unexpected side effects, be sure to let your doctor know so that alternatives can be considered.

Explore Professional Counseling

Professional counseling can help you any time some aspect of your life becomes overwhelming, your emotional problems become severe, or you want to prevent problems from getting worse. Certainly, any period of change can be made easier with the help of a support professional such as a psychiatrist, psychologist, social worker, psychiatric nurse, pastoral counselor, or another professional with the necessary credentials, compassion, and expertise.

Having somebody to talk to can be a big help, especially with a condition like prostate cancer. When you talk to your counselor, it may be one of the few times that you can be totally and brutally honest in releasing your feelings, and at the same time get feedback that can help you better deal with your feelings. Yes, it can be helpful to talk to family and friends and to other people in your situation. But none of these people may be able to provide you with the kind of frank intervention you can get from a therapist who is familiar with the feelings that exist when cancer enters your life. If you don't know an appropriate professional, you can get a referral from any of the physicians who are treating you, from the local chapter of the American Cancer Society, or from a local hospital.

Research has suggested that there are six different times in a person's experience with cancer when it might benefit him to discuss his feelings with a professional:

1. *At the time of diagnosis.* It is very common for individuals diagnosed with cancer to feel overwhelmed. Professional counseling can help you learn how to understand and accept the diagnosis, and to shift your focus to treatment so that you can learn how to help yourself.

2. *Before any treatment begins.* Prior to the beginning of treatment, professional help can prepare you for what lies ahead. And the better prepared you are, the more effective the treatment may be, and the greater control you'll have over your emotions.

3. *Following the onset of treatment.* Professionals can help you deal with any changes you experience at the beginning of treatment. You can discuss any side effects and prepare for anything that may occur as treatment continues.

4. *As treatment continues.* Throughout treatment, it's important to work through any feelings that develop. For example, if you've just had surgery, you may wonder if there will be any recurrences. Working with a professional at this time can help you maintain a positive attitude, and keep you committed to doing what you can to help yourself.

5. *After treatment is completed.* Once treatment is over, you may want to work with a professional to help keep your body and mind strong. You should focus on reestablishing new patterns of independence and reducing any dependence you may have on medical professionals.

6. *During the follow-up period.* As time goes on, it may be helpful to talk

to a professional and deal with any fears you have about the future, about recurrence, or about the need for additional treatment. You may also want to talk about any long-term side effects that may result from your treatment, as well as your concerns about returning to a more active lifestyle.

Obviously, it will be helpful to talk to professionals if the outcome is not what you want it to be. Fear of "things slipping away from you" is an important reason to speak to a professional. Counseling can help you get a grip on this slide, reverse it, and strengthen yourself for the future.

But not everyone needs professional help. Some people do very well on their own. So let's discuss some of the things you can do to better control your emotions.

Use Effective Coping Strategies

There are a number coping strategies you can use to better manage the emotions that may trouble you as you deal with prostate cancer. Any of these strategies can help you feel more in control and less depressed.

Make a conscious agreement with yourself. Tell yourself that you're going to set aside a little time each day to work on strengthening your emotional self and preparing yourself for the next day. During this special time, include activities such as relaxation, imagery, goal setting, or just positive thinking to improve your attitude. By consciously devoting time to this purpose, you will not only improve your overall emotional state, but will also give yourself an added feeling of control because you're doing something to help yourself.

Let's discuss some of the best techniques you can use to improve the way you feel.

Develop a Positive Mental Attitude

It is so important to have a positive mental attitude. Individuals with good mental attitudes are much better able to take control of their emotions. A negative mental attitude may exacerbate any emotional problems that occur because of, or in addition to, prostate cancer. So your primary goal should be to do all you can to improve your attitude in order to improve every other aspect of your life.

Concentrate on looking for the good. Why waste valuable time and energy focusing on the bad? You should always have hope. Hope is an integral part of the will to live. And research has clearly shown that the will to live plays an important part in the response to treatment.

The best source of hope is within yourself. You can always nurture hope based on what you hear from others. But hope has to start within. And this hope can remain strong as long as you're willing to do what you can to sustain yourself and fight for your life. A positive, optimistic attitude is very easy to cultivate, especially after you replace your initial pessimistic attitude.

Books may be very helpful in your efforts to generate a more positive mental attitude. There are many books in the library and in bookstores that offer suggestions for improving one's attitude. Look into some of these. If you get just one good idea out of a 300-page book, it will make the effort worthwhile.

Remember that this is your life we're talking about. You want to do whatever you can to maximize the positive aspects of your life. And improving your attitude is a very important part of that. If your attitude is positive, you'll feel better, regardless of what's going on around you. That's certainly worth the effort. Keep up your appearance, and try to be cheerful. Believe it or not, the act of *seeming* cheerful often leads to *feeling* cheerful. So walk tall and hold your head high. Feel good about who you are.

Laugh a Little

Laughter is one of the most effective coping strategies there is. Research has shown that the chemicals called *endorphins,* our own natural pain-killers, are released by the brain whenever we laugh. These endorphins can block pain and give us a feeling of well-being. Haven't you felt better—had a greater sense of well-being—after having a good laugh? You can enhance the process of getting better and staying better by building your sense of humor and making laughter an important part of your treatment program.

Humor is a pleasurable and effective way to deal with emotions. Whether you're listening to someone else's joke, laughing at yourself, or telling your own joke, humor can be a big help in troublesome situations. Now, you may be saying, "What's funny about prostate cancer?" Well, there may not *seem* to be anything funny about it, but you want to *find* funny things—both about the condition and about things in general—that will help you cope.

Humor works in three ways. First of all, it reduces anxiety. Laughter is one of the best ways known to release tension.

Second, laughter can distract you from those feelings or thoughts that are bothering you. When you're involved in something humorous, you often feel a lot better. Think back, for example, to a time when you were depressed or uncomfortable, and somebody asked if you had heard a certain joke. Initially, you may have been reluctant to hear it. But before long, you were probably totally absorbed in the joke, wondering what the punch line would be! The fact that humor can distract you also means that it can help you to see things from a different perspective. So you may be able to look at something more objectively—which can help you to handle it more effectively.

Finally, the ability to laugh at yourself is a helpful coping strategy. And it's an important part of maturing. How well this works, however, depends on what you're going through. It's just about impossible—and probably ridiculous—to laugh at yourself while you're going through a crisis. However, as you adjust to your condition, you will be able to better use humor as a coping strategy.

How can you make laughter-filled experiences a regular part of your everyday life? Watch funny things on television. Borrow videotapes that have funny movies or shows on them. Read funny books or magazines. Listen to comedy tapes. Read the comics. Any of these things can be incorporated into a program of helping yourself to have fun and feel better. Not only can these activities give you a quick boost by helping you distance yourself from anything that may be troubling you, but they can also improve your overall mood and physical well-being.

Set Goals for Yourself

Goal setting can be a very good way of coping with your emotions. What types of goals might you set? A good short-term goal might be the purchase of a new book by one of your favorite authors. A longer-term goal could involve the planning of a family vacation or activity, or, perhaps, a reunion of out-of-town friends. By setting realistic and positive goals—and working to realize them—you'll give yourself pleasurable events to look forward to, and a reason for getting through each and every day.

Be Nice to Yourself

Because you've been diagnosed with prostate cancer, you may feel that you've lost some control. You may even feel—incorrectly—that you're being punished.

It can be very helpful to offset these feelings by emphasizing the fact that nice things can happen to you. Often, it is important for individuals with chronic medical conditions to be just a little bit more "selfish"—that is, to initiate the kinds of activities or changes that will make them feel better. Of course, this should not be done in a way that is damaging to others. Instead, it should be done in a way that states repeatedly, "I am a worthwhile person, and I deserve to have nice things in my life."

Some people find it very difficult to learn how to be nice to themselves. Others may take it to the opposite extreme. They may be so-o-o nice to themselves that they have to temper their enthusiasm so as not to appear totally egocentric and self-centered!

What are some of the ways you can be nice to yourself? There are a number of different things you can do, such as buying yourself little goodies, giving yourself some special time to relax, involving yourself in favorite activities, spending more time with the people you enjoy, and so on. You may want to make a list of those things that would be most interesting and pleasurable for you. Everybody has the potential to do plenty of things that they enjoy.

Be Nice to Others

Sometimes, one of the best ways to boost your self-esteem is to be nice to other people. The feeling of pleasure you get from helping others can be very gratifying, and will very likely improve the way you feel about yourself.

What are some of the things you can do to be nice to others? You can help virtually any person in practically any aspect of his or her life, whether it is at home, at work, or at play. Visiting people in hospitals, nursing homes, and the like is one way to spread sunshine. Performing voluntary services in organizations such as churches, schools, and civic organizations is another possibility.

Helping others will make you feel better about yourself not only because you're performing a kind deed, but also because you're doing tangible things to better cope with your condition. You'll feel more productive. You'll feel more like you belong and are an important member of society. And, perhaps just as helpful, you'll find new ways of reducing boredom and channeling any excess energy or tension.

Derive Comfort From Faith

Individuals who have strong religious faith often find it very helpful in dealing with the emotions of cancer, and are able to derive a tremendous amount of solace from prayer. The religious beliefs of family and friends can also be a source of comfort to both you and them.

However, the degree to which people have faith varies, and the degree to which you exercise your religious beliefs are up to you. Don't feel that you *have* to turn to religion if this does not seem natural to you. Yet, if others have religious beliefs and you don't share their intensity, let them enjoy the comfort and support their faith provides for them, rather than questioning or mocking it.

Make Use of Relaxation Techniques

Relaxation is the opposite of tension. Therefore, if you learn to relax, you'll be much less tense! But relaxation procedures, by themselves, will not totally control your emotions. So why use them? Because if you're feeling more relaxed, you'll be better able to identify those problems that are affecting you and figure out how to deal with them. Relaxation procedures, then, can be an essential first step in coping with your emotions.

How can you relax? We're talking about clinical relaxation, now—not everyday activities like reading, gardening, listening to music, or sitting in front of the television with a can of beer! There are several different types of clinical relaxation procedures, including progressive relaxation, meditation, autogenics, deep breathing, and a technique that I call the Quick Release. All of these techniques are discussed in Chapter 19, along with imagery, hypnosis, and biofeedback—three techniques that can be used for a number of different reasons, including relaxation.

Remember that if you have difficulty learning to relax on your own, there's nothing wrong with seeking out a professional who can help you learn some of these skills.

Pinpoint What's Bothering You

Are you more comfortable now? Then you're ready to proceed to the next crucial step. In order to deal with anything that's upsetting you, you have to determine exactly what it is that's bothering you! Make a list of these things. Then go over what you've written. In reviewing your list, you'll see that just about every item can be placed into one of two categories. The first category contains the "modifiables"—the problems or emotions that you *can* do something about. The second category includes the "nonmodifiables"—the things you *can't* do anything about.

Why separate them? Because different strategies should be used to deal with these two types of problems.

For the first category, you'll want to figure out what techniques you can use to improve the situation. How about the second category? You'll still be planning strategies, but of a different kind! Where do your emotions exist? In your mind, right? Therefore, your plan for this category is to work on the way you're thinking.

Work on Your Thinking

How can you change your thinking so that something will bother you less? The technique you choose should depend on the specific emotional reaction that's bothering you. For example, if you're afraid of something and you want to conquer this fear, a procedure called systematic desensitization may be helpful. We'll go into this later in Chapter 12. Then again, if you're feeling guilty or angry about something, or if something is depressing you, it can be very helpful to learn how to change or "restructure" the way you're thinking. You'll learn more about techniques for that in Chapters 11, 13, and 14.

How do you deal with uncertainty? One of the first things to do is to focus on living as a person who happens to have cancer, rather than seeing yourself as a cancer victim. Try to enjoy life as much as possible. And try to live your life as normally as you can, doing as much as you normally would. Concentrate on what you have, not what you have not. Concentrate on what you can still do, not what you can no longer do. Emphasize the quality of your life, not the quantity. Focus on what you're going to do to make the most of every day. People who are successful are the ones who live life one day at a time, making the most of each day as they live it.

Actually, any of the techniques we've discussed can be used to cope with just about any problem. It's simply a question of deciding what works best for *you*.

WHAT ABOUT THE FUTURE?

Remember that you are the same person you were before you were diagnosed. The fact that you have prostate cancer doesn't mean that anything else about you has changed. Keep this in mind, and try to retain as much control over your life as you can. If there are ways in which you can improve your control, do so.

Even if you are now experiencing intense emotional reactions, be reassured that these feelings will diminish, either because of the passage of time or because you're doing something to help yourself. On the other hand, you can expect to experience more emotional reactions during those times when your symptoms are more pronounced. So you'll probably have a range of emotional reactions from time to time. But even when these feelings do occur, you will usually be able to point to so many positive things in your life—to so many ways in which you can recognize progress—that it may not be as difficult to deal with these feelings as you fear. In this way, you'll be able to develop the positive mental attitude that you want to become an integral part of your life.

The purpose of the following seven chapters is to help you understand the different emotions you may experience. You'll discover where these emotions come from, and recognize that many other individuals have gone through exactly what you're going through now. In addition, a number of strategies will be presented to help you cope with these emotions more effectively. Remember that "practice makes better." Just reading about a method used to control an emotion doesn't guarantee success. You have to keep practicing.

In the following chapters, you'll see how these different techniques can be used. So don't be afraid, depressed, angry, or guilty! Instead, read on!

Chapter 10

COPING WITH THE DIAGNOSIS

The diagnosis of prostate cancer can be devastating, regardless of where or how you hear it. You might hear it in the doctor's office, on the telephone, or even in the recovery room of the hospital following surgery. However, there's no easy way to accept the fact that this diagnosis means that your life is going to change.

INITIAL REACTIONS

When first diagnosed, some people may not even react, since it may not be "real" to them. But others go through a hard time from the very beginning. It's shocking to be told that you have cancer. It can stun you. You may immediately feel separated from your emotions—that what's going on is unreal.

Most people who are diagnosed with cancer are scared—scared of dying, scared of pain, scared of rejection, scared of isolation. These feelings are very common. Right after you have been told that you have cancer, it is virtually impossible to think straight about what you're going to do in the future—about treatment, prognosis, changes in lifestyle, or anything else.

You may know someone who has prostate cancer, or you may have heard about the experiences of some people who've had it. This may frighten you even more. Emotional reactions to prostate cancer are not always rational. As a matter of fact, in many cases they are completely irrational. And as the full impact of the diagnosis sets in, you may experience a whole variety of feelings ranging from sadness and anxiety to anger, frustration, and despair.

Some people react to the diagnosis of prostate cancer in a very volatile, angry way. Others are superficially calm. But who knows what emotions they are bottling up inside, and when those emotions will be expressed?

You may be surprised to hear that a percentage of people—a *small* percentage of people—are relieved when they're diagnosed with prostate cancer. (Yes, relieved!) Why? Because at least now they know what the problem is so that, hopefully, treatment can cure, or at least stop the progression of, the disease. Most people, however, experience a much more frightening, intense, panicky reaction. Let's look in greater detail at some of the more common reactions to diagnosis. Later in the chapter, we'll look at how you can begin to cope with these emotions.

Panic!

Immediately after diagnosis, the most commonly experienced reaction—and certainly not a pleasant one—is terror. Sheer panic! You may think, "Oh, no, I have cancer! Where did it come from? Why do I have it?" Or you may ask, "What's going to happen to me?" "How will prostate cancer affect me?" "What is the treatment (and how will I handle it)?" "Will I ever get better?" "Who will take care of me?" "Am I going to die?" You may think that your life will never be the same again, because life will now include prostate cancer. And family members and loved ones may have the same fears and ask the same questions—and they, too, may panic.

Let's talk about this reaction. Does anyone you know like having cancer? No way. It's normal to be upset and afraid. You probably didn't understand the diagnosis at first. After all, how much did you know about prostate cancer beforehand? Just the word cancer is frightening!

You may suddenly be hit with the fact that you are mortal and vulnerable. You may start fearing for your life! Physically, it's not uncommon to feel faint or dizzy, or to experience other stress reactions at the time of diagnosis.

Because of the tremendous fears that can immediately follow diagnosis—fears of loss of health, loss of income, loss of love, and possibly even loss of life—it's not surprising that the time following diagnosis is one of turmoil. The path to recovering from this turmoil is rarely smooth. A whole other group of emotions, such as rage, anger, depression, and fear, comes into play.

All of these emotions don't occur just in you. They occur also in your family members who, along with sharing the other concerns you may have, may feel helpless because they don't know what they can do for you. This can certainly make things worse—for them *and* for you.

Although it may take you a long time to accept the reality of the diagnosis, the process of acceptance began the moment the diagnosis was heard. Unfortunately, acceptance must take place. What other choice do you have?!

Shock and Disbelief

Disbelief is a very common reaction of people diagnosed with cancer. You may feel that this can't be happening to you—that someone must have made a mistake. This disbelief can last for hours. For some people, it can last for days or even weeks.

The initial feeling of disbelief eventually gives way to a feeling of numbness. You may sit transfixed, staring into space, not really hearing what's going on. You may hear your doctor talking, even hear the reassuring words, but his words will not penetrate. You may even calmly participate in the discussion without showing any emotions. (Those may come later!) However, be aware that this numbness serves as insulation. It helps to keep you from falling apart, and allows you to begin accepting the diagnosis at your own rate.

Denial

As we've already discussed, it's not at all unusual to deny that a problem exists. Regardless of the symptoms you've been experiencing, hearing that you have prostate cancer may provoke denial. You may protest, "Oh, you're just making that up," "I don't have this problem," "Why don't you give it a little more time? I'm sure the problem will go away by itself," or even, "#!(*) x#, leave me alone!"

If you're reading this book, chances are you're probably not denying your condition. But if you are denying, somewhere along the line you're going to have to start facing reality. How? Speak to professionals who know about prostate cancer, and have them explain it in further detail. Let them tell you about the available treatments for your condition. Read about prostate cancer. Or talk to other people with prostate cancer, and listen to what they went through when they were first diagnosed. You will find that many of their experiences parallel your own. You'll also find that many of them have learned to adjust—just as you'll eventually adjust!

Do you ever ask yourself, "Why can't I go back to the way things used to be?" Do you ever wish you could wake up one morning and find out that this was all a bad dream? The more you keep hoping that the situation will go away, the more you will slow down your adjustment. Why? Because you're not really admitting to yourself that you've changed, perhaps permanently. Rather, you're trying to push it out of your mind, hoping that things will return to the way they were. Try to recognize that your condition does exist now, that it affects you, and that it will remain with you. Then aim your efforts in the *right* direction. Try to plan all your activities and structure all your thinking towards handling your situation as effectively as you can.

HOW CAN YOU BEGIN TO ADJUST?

You may have many questions immediately following your diagnosis. However, the most important question is the one that only you can answer. And that question is, "Will I give up living because of cancer, or will I continue to live despite cancer?" The following steps should start you on the path to living successfully with prostate cancer.

Take Charge

You must take the reins and begin to help yourself. Sure, you can receive love and support from your family and friends, and you can get guidance and expertise from professionals. But that's never enough. You are the one who is going to have to come to grips with prostate cancer. At first, adjusting may be a difficult struggle that requires a tremendous effort. You may go through a lot of emotional turmoil. But there is no other way out. You must face it.

Information, Please!

Many of your initial reactions were probably the result of not knowing enough about prostate cancer. So you'll want to learn as much as possible. Your physician should be helpful in suggesting ways of getting current information.

It's very easy to let your imagination run wild. Initially, you'll probably keep thinking about all the things that can possibly go wrong. You'll worry about every symptom. You may also get frightened about how serious prostate cancer might get, and how it might affect you and the people close to you. So learn the facts about your condition. This is a great way to alleviate some of the anxiety caused by the diagnosis.

After reading general consumer-oriented information, you might want to move on to more technical material. Ask questions of your doctor about anything you don't understand. And certainly ask questions about anything that frightens you. After all, medical writing is not designed to calm the person with prostate cancer. It just states medical facts and statistics. Don't forget this, or you may get unnecessarily alarmed!

It probably wasn't a lifelong goal of yours to become an expert on prostate cancer, but think about how much this information may help you. Doctors will respect your questions more. And you'll understand exactly what's going on in your body. These are just two of the many advantages that can come from reading about your condition.

When people first find out about your diagnosis, many will probably send you additional information about prostate cancer and its treatment, or try to share stories about others with prostate cancer. Sure, there are times when this can be helpful, but make sure that the information you receive is reputable. And if you find you're receiving too much information, you may want to designate certain members of your family or close friends to be intermediaries for you. Let them go through all the material, find anything that might be important, and share these facts with you. This may do a lot to eliminate the stress in your life.

Certainly, many valuable facts about cancer can be obtained from the Cancer Information Service, an organization maintained by the National Cancer Institute. Don't hesitate to call the institute's toll-free telephone number (1-800-4-CANCER) and tell them what kind of information you're looking for so that they can provide you with helpful materials.

You may also want to contact organizations such as the American Cancer Society or Cancer Care. These and other groups may be located in your area, or you may be able to call national offices to get as much up-to-date information as possible. (See the resource list on page 279 for details.)

Begin Facing Your Fears

Once you've accepted the fact that you have prostate cancer, you can start determining what changes you may have to make in your lifestyle. In addition, you'll want to try to control as many harmful emotions as you can.

The emotions stemming from the diagnosis of prostate cancer can be unpleasant. You may experience regret, sorrow, and nostalgia, remembering the way life used to be. Many fears may come to mind, some of which may be overwhelming. Fears of incapacitation, of death, and of losing friends are all very common. Begin facing them. They can and must be faced in order to move your adjustment along more smoothly. Speak to other people who have prostate cancer. Learn how they've adjusted. This can be very helpful.

Develop a Positive Relationship With Your Doctor

Obviously, you must work with a physician you can trust, one who has had experience working with people with prostate cancer. As stated earlier in the chapter, you have the right—in fact, the obligation—to learn as much as possible about the different treatments for prostate cancer. And you can start by asking questions of your physician. Remember that the patient-physician relationship is very important in the case of prostate cancer, as it is with any chronic illness. If your physician does not seem receptive to your questions, try to discuss how important these questions are to you. If no progress is made, then you may have to reconsider this relationship and look for another care provider.

Because your medical problem will be ongoing, your relationship with your physician will be ongoing as well. You will have much more contact with your physician than you would if you didn't have prostate cancer. In fact, some say that this relationship is like a marriage—although, unfortunately, you won't be entitled to 50 percent of your doctor's assets if you separate!

Help Your Family Adjust

It is understandably difficult to adjust to the diagnosis of cancer and cope with the different emotions you are experiencing. This adjustment becomes that much harder when the people close to you also have difficulty with their emotions—especially if their emotions are different from yours!

Of course, it's easy to understand why family members might have trouble dealing with the diagnosis. They, too, will go through periods of denial—times during which they'll say, "No, everything will be fine," or, "I'm sure the problem will clear up by itself." Unfortunately, this won't make things easier for you.

Bill, a teacher, was sixty years old when he was diagnosed as having prostate cancer. After a couple of very depressing months, Bill started to learn how to cope. He was finally able to handle thoughts of lifestyle changes, concerns about reduced energy, and some of the other unpleasant realities associated with his condition. Sound great? Not really. You see, Bill's wife of thirty-eight years couldn't accept the fact that he had this problem, his children were afraid he was going to die, and his fifty-eight-year-old brother had contacted virtually every cancer specialist from New York to Alaska! Although Bill was learning how to cope with prostate cancer, he could not cope with his family. They couldn't handle it, and were making things very difficult for him.

It's a great idea for family members to seek out people to speak to—just as it may benefit *you* to seek help. Spouses, children, and others can find out more about prostate cancer and learn how others cope with ti ..tment. They can even join support groups or seek counseling. So encourage your family and any willing friends to learn as much as they can and to seek whatever help they need. Their adjustment will help your adjustment.

SUMMING UP

Start thinking positively about your life with prostate cancer. Learn as much as you can about your condition. Use whatever support systems are necessary. Use all the stress-management and emotional-control techniques you can learn. (Many good ones can be found in this book!) Start saying to yourself, "Prostate cancer may be a part of my life, but I'm still alive, and I'm going to do whatever I can to help myself adjust to this."

If it's necessary for you to make changes in your lifestyle, even major ones, tell yourself that you will make them, and that you will make them willingly! You're going to lead as complete a life as you can. The more quickly you can adjust your lifestyle to fit your needs, the more rapidly you'll be able to enjoy your life. This may be hard at first, and certainly will take time. But you can be grateful that you're not helpless, and that you can take steps to make the most of your life despite prostate cancer!

Chapter 11

DEPRESSION

Albert was feeling very down. A sixty-five-year-old father of four, married for twenty-nine years, living in a comfortable home in a good neighborhood, he apparently had everything he could ask for. But he certainly hadn't asked for prostate cancer! He found himself feeling increasingly upset with the changes that had to be made in his life. He was getting tired too easily. He was afraid that his life would be shorter. He didn't have enough energy for his family. He felt helpless and hopeless. In short, Albert was suffering from depression.

Depression is a serious problem. The very mention of the word can sometimes knock the smile right off your face. Actual numbers vary, but it is estimated that at least 5 million Americans need professional care for depression. Because it is so widespread, depression has been nick-named the "common cold" of emotional problems.

Just what is depression? Depression is an extremely unpleasant feeling of unhappiness and despair. It can range from a mild problem—feeling discouraged and downhearted—to a severe disorder—feeling utterly hopeless, worthless, and unwilling to go on living. You may believe that there is no reason to remain a part of the world. You may be afraid of being a burden to your family, and think that everybody would be better off without you. Or you may just feel useless.

Depression can be painful. Imagine how it must hurt to feel (or say), "I wish I were never born. What good am I? I'm not helping anybody around me, and I'm not helping myself." It may seem as if the world is against you. Life may seem unfair—a constant struggle in which you never win. And that hurts.

Family members, too, can suffer from depression. This may result from a number of things, including lifestyle changes. In many cases, this problem may go unnoticed by others, and so may go untreated. And the troubled family members may feel very guilty about their problem. Why? They may think that since they're not the ones who are sick, they don't have a right to be upset!

WHAT ARE THE SYMPTOMS OF DEPRESSION?

There are a number of possible symptoms of depression. If you notice that you're feeling excessive amounts of sadness, despair, discouragement, or melancholy; if you're unable to eat, and this problem has nothing to do with the cancer or its treatment; if you're sleeping either too much or too little; if you feel totally withdrawn from social activities; if you find yourself crying, and that's not typical behavior for you; if you're brooding about the past and feeling hopeless—any of these feelings may indicate depression. And there are other symptoms of depression, as well. If you're experiencing excessive amounts of irritability or anger; if your fears seem to be extreme; if you feel inadequate and worthless; if you are unable to concentrate on virtually anything in your life, whether it be work, family, or other interests; if you seem to have little or no interest in activities that previously gave you pleasure; if you have reduced amounts of energy that don't seem to be related to disease or treatment; if you have little or no interest in sex or intimacy; and if your cognitive style (the way you speak, think, and act) seems to be generally slowing down—these, too, can be symptomatic of depression. The more of these symptoms you are experiencing, the more likely it is that you are depressed and should take some action to help yourself.

HOW DOES DEPRESSION AFFECT YOU?

Now you know some of the many possible symptoms of depression. But the effects of depression are not isolated problems. Depression can affect your physical well-being, can take control of your moods, and can make it difficult to enjoy—or even carry out—the simplest activity. Let's take a look at some of the ways that depression can affect you in your day-to-day life.

How Depression Affects Your Body

Some of the more noticeable symptoms of depression are physical in nature. Nervous activity or agitation, such as wringing of the hands, may occur. You may be restless or have difficulty remaining in one place. Or, on the other hand, you may become much less active and remain motionless for abnormally long periods of time, appearing to be almost in a trance, with no apparent desire or energy to do anything.

If you're depressed, most of your physical activities will also slow down—and not just because of physical limitations. You're probably feeling exhausted. This may be surprising, since you're not doing much of anything. But constantly telling yourself that you're no good can be very tiring! You really don't want to believe this, but you feel like you have no choice. And in attempting to escape from these feelings, you may become even more depressed, as well as more physically drained and exhausted.

Depression may also cause you to feel physically sick, or to experience a reduction or increase in appetite. Of course, it's wise to remember that any of these symptoms might be related to a physical disorder. So even if the symptoms go away when your depression improves, don't just assume that they're related to the depression. A medical examination may still be a good idea. This way, you'll be sure that there is no organic cause for your depression.

How Depression Affects Your Moods and Outlook

If you're depressed, you may experience frequent mood swings. For example, you might feel worse in the morning and better in the evening. This nightly improvement may occur because each evening you realize that it's almost time to go to sleep—to escape. But depression may also cause difficulty in sleeping, even if you weren't doing much of anything during the day. If you're mildly depressed, you may have difficulty concentrating, and your attention span may be much shorter. When you speak, your conversation may emphasize feelings of worthlessness and despair.

When you're depressed, it's typical to feel as if your mood keeps getting lower. You like yourself very little, if at all. Your thinking is very negative, very different from the way it was when you were feeling good. In fact, it is this negative thinking—not just a particular triggering event—that leads to depression. (But more on this later in the chapter.)

Naturally, your day-to-day activities may suffer as a result of these negative feelings. You may, for instance, remain unshaven simply because you don't feel like shaving. Or you may "go through the motions" of your everyday activities, even though your heart isn't in them. Many people, in fact, simply withdraw from their usual activities during bouts of depression.

How Depression Affects Relationships With Others

Do you now feel less at ease talking to others? Does it seem like others are having a hard time talking to you, even if they have been close to you for a long time? As already discussed, because of your depression, you may be less interested in conversation, and you may feel less confident. You may project your negative feelings about yourself onto others, and believe that they really don't want to talk to you. And the more depressed you become, the better you may get at convincing the people around you that you're no good. You may feel that others have no need for you. You may feel that they consider you to be an uninteresting, boring person.

Pete received a telephone call from his friend Joe. Joe wanted to know how Pete had been feeling, since the last time they had gotten together, Pete had seemed very tired. Pete responded halfheartedly, imagining that Joe was calling only out of obligation. He then explained that he would understand if Joe did not want to call again, since he never seemed to have any good news to tell him. How do you think Joe felt? Imagine hearing this repeatedly! Would you be surprised if, eventually, Joe got tired of even trying, and simply stopped calling? But in Pete's mind, this would only reinforce his feelings that he really was no good—that he was not worthy of having any friends after all!

WHAT CAUSES DEPRESSION?

A bout of depression frequently seems to start with one specific thing— one upsetting event or occurrence. Gene had been planning a trip to see his grandchildren for over two months. Although he had been more tired recently, he still was able to buy gifts for his grandchildren, and looked forward to seeing their reaction to the presents. In the weeks prior to the trip, Gene tried to get as much rest as possible. The day of his trip finally came. But Gene felt so physically weak that his doctor told him he couldn't make the trip. That one disappointment triggered a long depression. Gene felt like the most important things in his life were being ruined by his prostate cancer.

What happens after the first depressing event occurs? A kind of chain reaction can follow. This one occurrence may create a feeling that spreads like wildfire. It's almost as if the bottom has dropped out of your world. You may feel that you are less able to control your thinking—although this is not true, as we will see later in this chapter.

Still, a disappointing or upsetting event doesn't *always* lead to depression. So where does depression come from, and why does it sometimes take hold? Sometimes we can figure this out, and sometimes we can't. But before we give up, let's discuss some of the possible causes.

How About the "Normal Downs"?

A certain amount of depression is normal in anyone's life. We all experience normal cycles of ups and downs. If we never experienced some of the downs, how could we fully appreciate the ups!? However, when depression becomes more than just the "normal downs," it must be attended to. Nipping it quickly in the bud can keep it from becoming much worse.

Of course, certain events—traumatic experiences such as losing a loved one, being diagnosed with a chronic medical problem, requiring major surgery, or being fired from a job—can lead anyone into a depression. However, the fact that the cause is understandable doesn't mean that you should ignore the problem or wait until it goes away. It's necessary to learn how to deal with depression, as this is an essential part of coping with prostate cancer.

How About Anger You Can't Express?

What if you get so angry that you feel like you're going to burst? But you don't—or can't—do anything about it, so you decide to "swallow" your anger. It seems strange that a powerful feeling like anger can turn into a withdrawn, helpless feeling like depression. But it can. If you become increasingly angry about something and feel unable to do anything about it, you may turn the anger inward. You may feel so much frustration or hopelessness that you "shut down" in an attempt to keep yourself from experiencing these terrible feelings. This leads to withdrawal, which is a symptom of depression. (For more information on anger, see Chapter 13.)

Could It Be a Chemical Imbalance?

In a small percentage of cases, depression may be caused by biochemical deficiencies—chemical imbalances in our bodies. This does not occur very often, however. Treatment for biochemical deficiencies may involve the administration of drugs in an effort to rebalance body chemistry. (See Chapter 18 for information on antidepressants.) This usually isn't the whole answer. But regardless of whether your depression is caused by this or, more typically, by your reactions to the people and events around you, you should still try to modify your thinking. Many experts believe that even if the cause of depression is biochemical, by working on the way you handle your day-to-day living, you can have a positive effect on your depression.

How About Prostate Cancer?

Can prostate cancer cause depression? Are you kidding??? The seriousness of the condition can certainly either create depression or magnify already-existing depression. So it is not surprising that a certain degree of depression can almost be expected if you are living with cancer. Depression often starts immediately after the diagnosis, lasts for a while, and then reappears from time to time during the course of treatment. This is totally normal.

What contributes to depression in people with cancer? One contributor is an unsatisfied need for control. Most people have the need to be in control of at least certain aspects of their life, and cancer can quickly make you feel out of control. It is realistic to admit to yourself that you may not be in control of everything at this point. There may be certain things that are beyond your reach. However, it is also realistic to recognize that you can still control certain things, and that it is better to focus your energy in this direction.

Related to this unsatisfied need for control is a feeling of helplessness. Before the diagnosis, you may have felt strong and self-reliant. Now, however, you may feel weak, uncertain about the future, and powerless to help yourself. This can certainly lead to depression.

Another contributor to depression can be an unwillingness to mourn the lost sense of immortality that comes with a chronic illness. You may feel that it's simply not your style to grieve. If so, you're practicing a type of denial that takes such excessive amounts of energy to maintain that depression may result.

What else about prostate cancer may depress you? You may become depressed thinking about the future, wondering how prostate cancer will affect your life. You may get depressed as a result of the treatment for your cancer. Problems involving other people may depress you, too. You may feel helpless at not being able to share what you're experiencing. You may get depressed if others don't understand what you're going through—not that you want to be pitied, though! People may expect more from you than you're able or willing to provide. You may be depressed over the possibility of damaged relationships, lost friendships, or family friction. If you're single, you may become depressed thinking that this will affect possible relationships—not that there need be any truth to this at all!

Depression may also result from changes in lifestyle. You may not be able to participate in the activities you used to love. You may have to change your work routine, as well as your family routine. Money problems, with no immediate solution in sight, can certainly be depressing. Just having prostate cancer, with its intangible effects on your day-to-day living, can get to you.

You may be saying to yourself, "If I'm depressed over my prostate cancer, how can I expect to get over my depression unless my prostate cancer is cured?" This kind of thinking will get you nowhere. You don't want your emotional state to depend on your physical state. So if your depression lingers, don't wait. Work on it. Learn how to cope with it. Later, we'll talk more later about how you can improve your thinking.

WHAT MAINTAINS DEPRESSION?

If you're depressed, you may be blaming yourself—or your prostate cancer—for everything that is wrong. You may tend to become more and more withdrawn, and pull away from the world around you. Why? Well, if you believe that your condition is causing all these horrible things, isn't it better to "escape" and not think about it? Realistically, escaping won't solve anything. But you may feel that withdrawal is the only way to stop feeling terrible. And this will keep you depressed. (In fact, it may make you even more depressed.)

Although you may seem sullen and withdrawn to others, you're probably in deep emotional pain. And part of what is making you, and keeping you, depressed is your effort to protect yourself from this emotional pain. You feel that nothing good can possibly happen—that only bad things can happen. So what do you do? You try to block everything out of your mind!

So why do you stay depressed? Why doesn't it just go away? It may be because you don't want to talk to anybody, or to even consider counseling. Therefore, the thoughts and feelings that lead to your depression have been kept hidden. You may ask, "Is my unwillingness to talk the only reason I'm still depressed? If I start talking more, will that get me out of my depression?" Not necessarily. But it can be helpful to talk out your feelings. It would probably be beneficial—even though you wouldn't be too thrilled—if a close friend or family member took the initiative and forced you into some kind of conversation, therapeutic or otherwise, or, at least, pushed you into doing something constructive.

HOW CAN YOU COPE WITH DEPRESSION?

Can anything be done to end depression? Of course! Would I abandon you without any suggestions? First, tell yourself that the main reason you're depressed is that you haven't yet taken the proper steps toward feeling better! These steps can pull you out of your rut and reacquaint you with the more positive, pleasant aspects of living—the aspects that you'd like to experience.

Don't think it will be easy, though. Unfortunately, once you've fallen into depression, it takes hard work and a certain amount of persistence to pull yourself back out. The result, however, is surely worth the fight.

And, of course, the fight will be easier if you know of specific techniques and activities that will help.

Because you have prostate cancer, it is inevitable that you will experience some depression. Don't be afraid of it. Rather, expect it and prepare yourself for it. This will help you better deal with depression when it does occur.

Once you feel better, you're not going to ever want to feel depressed again, right? Well, the strategies and techniques that are most effective in dealing with depression can also be effective in preventing you from becoming depressed again, but, unfortunately, this doesn't mean that you'll never again feel depressed. It may happen. Anticipate it, so that if it does recur, you won't completely fall apart. And if this feeling does come back, won't it be good to know that you *can* do something to help yourself?

One of the first things that you must do in learning to cope with depression is to accept the limitations in your life. Accept the fact that you can't control *everything* around you or become involved in *everything*. This does not mean that you are powerless, but it does mean that you may have to alter your views about what you can and can't do. Once you accept your limitations, you'll be able to focus your energy in appropriate, constructive directions instead of lamenting what has changed. How can you accept your limitations? Well, let's say that you were previously able to do twenty-five things in your life, and now, because of prostate cancer, you're not able to do twenty-three of them. Instead of wasting your energy thinking about the twenty-three things you can no longer do, focus your energy on feeling good about the two things you can do. Remember the Serenity Prayer: "Lord, grant me the serenity to accept the things I cannot change, the courage to change the things I can, and the wisdom to know the difference."

Another strategy you can use to alleviate depression is to exercise choice. Demonstrating that you have the ability to choose certain things in your life will help increase your feeling of control. Sure, there may be certain events that are beyond your control. But you can still focus your energy on all those things that you can do.

Regardless of what you have to do and what mountains seem to stand in your way, the most you can ask of yourself—the most that anybody can ask of himself or herself—is to take one step at a time. Just keep taking one more step. This will be helpful, especially if you're feeling overwhelmed because there are so many things to do.

Now that you're ready to fight your depression, consider two major ways of dealing with it: being more physical (in other words, doing something), and working on your thinking. It can be very helpful to make a list of all the things that are depressing you. You may feel that there will be at least fifty items! But, in actuality, you'll probably start running out of ideas after six or seven. Then divide this list into two more lists: first, the things you can do something about, and second, the things you can't do anything about. (Sound familiar? Sure, you read about this earlier. But it works for a number of different problems.) Get physical— do something—about those items in the first list; and get thoughtful— work on your thinking—regarding those items in the second list.

Let's Get Physical

There are two ways of getting physical in order to deal with depression: actively working to accomplish goals, and increasing physical activity. Hopefully, as suggested above, you've listed all the things that are depressing you, and have made a separate list of those items that can be changed. Now think about ways in which you can modify or eliminate the items on this list. Be realistic but aggressive in planning ways to reach your goals—even if it can't be done all at once.

Where does the physical activity come in? Unknowingly, you may be using a lot of energy to keep yourself depressed. You may be working hard to keep that anger inside, even if it appears to others that you're simply withdrawing. If your depression is anger turned within, we can logically assume that by releasing your anger, you'll be able to eliminate your feelings of depression. But what should you do with those feelings? You must find an object towards which your anger can be expressed. This may be difficult. However, it's important to release the trapped anger so that it doesn't build up further and deepen the depression.

Think about the following situation. You're sitting there, depressed and withdrawn. Somebody makes an innocent remark, and you practically bite the person's head off! What's happening? Whatever was said triggered the release of the internalized anger that was making you depressed. Look out, world!

What kinds of activities can help you release your anger? Many physical activities can be effective. Try walking, playing golf or tennis, or swimming. Whatever activity you choose, though, be sure to get your doctor's okay before beginning your exercise program. (For more information on exercise, see Chapter 22.)

Let's Get Thoughtful

Although getting physical may help lift your depression—and can also provide a great distraction, which may help you to look more objectively at what's going on—physical activity will not teach you ways of fighting inappropriate thinking. Remember that it's your *thoughts* that have made you depressed. Clearly, restructuring your thinking is a key element in alleviating depression and dealing with any negative emotions.

If you can "think" yourself into depression, obviously, you can also "think" yourself out of it. How? If you're depressed, you're just talking yourself *down*. All your comments—or at least most of them—are probably put-downs: harsh statements that can make you feel even worse. You want your inner voice to help you, not hurt you. Let's see how you can do that.

Distinguish Fact From Fiction

Don't get defensive when I tell you this, but when you're depressed, you tend to distort reality. Clinical research with depressed patients has proven this. Recognize, therefore, that your thoughts are not necessarily based on what is truly happening, but, instead, may be based on your own distorted views. This is called *cognitive distortion.*

Is that bad? You bet your happiness it is! "Cognitive" refers to your thinking. "Distortion" means you're twisting things around and, in general, losing sight of what's real. We all tend to do this from time to time. But when you're depressed, you do it a lot, if not all the time, and it keeps you depressed. So how do you stop? First, you must become reacquainted with what is really happening—with the facts. But how can you do that if you keep distorting reality? Right now, you're better off accepting somebody else's perceptions of the situation, because that person is probably a lot more objective and accurate. Since so many feelings of worthlessness are based on distorted facts, depression can be reduced, if not eliminated, once these facts have been straightened out.

Sam kept moaning because none of his friends were calling him. "They don't call as much as they used to. I guess they just don't care." His sister, Sue, asked him to estimate how often his friends used to call. When Sam compared this number with the current number of calls he was receiving, he realized that the numbers were almost the same. He then recognized that he was probably just more sensitive because of all the changes going on in his life! Although he did not feel 100-percent better, Sam did feel a good deal better, because he could now see that he hadn't been abandoned.

So make sure you know what true and what's not. Ask yourself for your own assessment of the situation, and be as objective as possible. Then, if necessary, ask other people—people whose opinions you trust—for their evaluation. Work to become more comfortable with any differences in perception and to adjust your thinking so that it more closely matches the actual circumstances.

Make Molehills Out of Mountains

Does this imply that if you're depressed you have no real problem? Is it "all in your head"? No. Everyone has problems. If you feel good, you can handle them; but if you're depressed, you may feel overwhelmed—each and every obstacle and task, regardless of how trivial or slight it may be, will tend to depress you.

Again, do your best to view each problem objectively—to avoid blowing it out of proportion. Eventually, as your depression lifts, you will be able to deal with all of life's problems, big and small.

Avoid Self-Fulfilling Prophecies

We've discussed several thoughts that are characteristic of depression—thoughts that you may be having right now. Are all these thoughts and feelings irrational and untrue? No. But, ironically, although some of them may start off being far from the truth, the longer you feel this way, the greater the chance that they will become self-fulfilling prophecies. In other words, the more you allow yourself to think negatively, the greater the likelihood that your fears will turn into realities. For example, if you begin telling yourself that friends and relatives don't care, this may become a reality, because your negative attitude may alienate the people close to you. And if you feel less able or less willing to do the things you used to do, your inactivity is likely to magnify and confirm your feelings of worthlessness, leading to even greater depression and helplessness. Not a pretty picture.

Once you begin feeling depressed, your negative thoughts will soon lead to negative actions. These negative actions will lead to more negative thoughts, which will in turn lead to more negative actions, and so on. It is an ongoing, vicious cycle that will spiral you further downward into deeper depression. Eventually you'll feel trapped in this vicious cycle, with no way to escape.

Are you getting depressed just reading this? In all probability, if you've ever been depressed, you've already said to yourself, "Wow, that sounds just like me!" So if you find that you're starting to believe in your negative thoughts, stop yourself. As we've said before, depression both results from and causes a lot of negative thinking. But once you become aware of these thoughts, you can do something about them. People who remain depressed feel incapable of doing anything about their negative thinking, and allow these thoughts to pull them into that vicious cycle mentioned earlier. Try to think positive thoughts, so that if one of your thoughts does turn into a reality, it will at least be a positive one.

Dwell on the Brighter Tomorrows

Mario was depressed because he constantly compared his present way of life with the way he had lived before his diagnosis of prostate cancer. Mario was afraid to swim (an activity that he loved), to stay out late with friends, to spend leisurely afternoons in museums, or to participate in other favorite activities. He allowed his depressing thoughts to overwhelm him, and, as a result, he certainly did not give himself a chance to enjoy life.

If you find yourself thinking along the same lines as Mario, try to modify your thoughts. Start planning fun things for the present and future. Anyone can come up with some enjoyable activities, regardless of physical restrictions. But it takes effort. Don't wallow in self-pity, because that will allow your depression to overwhelm you. Develop some positive plans, and translate them into pleasure. Then wave goodbye to your depression!

Of course, if you clearly reflect on your past, you may find that it wasn't much better than the present! In the past, you may have had other physical problems. You may have made some mistakes. Naturally, this may make you even more depressed about the future. However, you can't change the past. What's done is done. Keep telling yourself that. Don't punish yourself for the past. Tell yourself that you're going to work on making the future better. Set up some specific goals, starting with the easy-to-reach ones. You'll be helping yourself just by *thinking* about all the positive things you can do!

Rediscover What's Missing From Your Life

You may have laughed when you read the title of this section. "I *know* what's missing from my life," you might respond. "Good health. A cancer-free prostate!" Sure. But another important element that might very well be missing—an element that *can* be regained!—is the feeling of satisfaction, accomplishment, and pride that normally comes from others' praise. You may be missing the attention and interest of other people, and this may cause you to feel worthless. What can you do about this? Think about your positive qualities. (Yes, you do have some!) Think about how you can interact more with people, spark their interest, and obtain more of the satisfaction that makes you feel worthy.

Shoot for the Earth, Not the Moon

We all have goals for ourselves. It's normal to become depressed when we don't reach a particular goal, especially if we've tried very hard to get there. But sometimes our goal is not a realistic one.

Try to judge if the goals you've been setting for yourself are realistic. If not, reset your goals, with your abilities and limitations in mind. Once your goals are more realistic, you'll have a much better chance of achieving them, and less of a chance of falling short.

Talk About It!

Now you know how you can cope with depression both through physical activity and through changing your way of thinking. But there's one more thing you can do—something we've mentioned before. You can *talk* about your problems and concerns with others. Often, the very act of talking will help lift your depression. And whom should you talk to? If there are family members or friends whom you feel close to and whose opinions you trust, talk to them. Air your feelings, and listen to their feedback. They may be more objective than you at this time, and may be better able to come up with constructive solutions.

If your depression is so intense or prolonged that friends and family are unable to help, then by all means consider speaking to a professional. Counseling has an increasingly effective reputation for treating depression. Don't deny yourself this invaluable assistance. Why not do everything you can to help yourself feel better?

AN ANTI-DEPRESSING SUMMARY

The best way to work on negative thoughts is to prevent them from continuing. Be realistically positive. Deal with reality the way it actually exists. Deal with thoughts from a more factual point of view. Handle them the way they might be handled by somebody else—somebody who is not depressed and who can be more objective. Try to make your perceptions more accurate, your awareness more realistic, and your thoughts more constructive. Remember: Your thoughts lead to your emotions. If your thoughts are negative and critical, your emotions will also be in bad shape. If you can turn your thoughts around to a more positive, constructive point of view, your emotional reactions will most certainly follow. And depression will then be a thing of the past.

Chapter 12

FEARS AND ANXIETIES

Don't be *afraid* to read this chapter! It may help you discover what you're *anxious* about!

The two sentences above may help you to distinguish between fear and anxiety. What is the difference? Anxiety is a general sense of uneasiness: a vague feeling of discomfort. It is an agitated, uncertain state in which you just don't feel at peace or in control. There is a premonition that something bad may happen—something you have to protect yourself against. You feel very vulnerable. However, you're not exactly sure what the source of your anxiety is.

Fear, on the other hand, is usually more specific. It's often directed toward something that can be recognized, whether a person, an object, a situation, or an event. We have fear when we become aware of something dangerous, or when we feel threatened. When we are afraid—much like when we're anxious—we feel out of control and less confident. So the feelings of fear and anxiety are basically the same, the main difference being whether the source of the feeling can be identified. Moreover, the strategies used to combat fear will also enable you to cope with anxiety. For this reason, from this point on, we'll be using the two terms interchangeably.

Fear is so common that we have developed a number of different words to describe it: scared, concerned, alarmed, worried, nervous, and edgy. Then there's wary, frightened, and helpless. Is that it? Nope! How about suspicious, keyed-up, hesitant, apprehensive, tense, panicky, disturbed, and agitated? Of course, there are more, but if I continued, this book would have to be renamed *The Fear Synonym Book*. The point is that all these words mean the same thing: "I'm afraid." The source of this fear may be real or imaginary.

FEAR AND PROSTATE CANCER

Fear can hit you the instant you first hear the word "cancer." Fear can hit you the first time a doctor tells you that the cancer is affecting your prostate gland. So many fears may circulate in your mind that you may feel overwhelmed. You may be fearful that you're going to need surgery. You may be fearful of the unknown.

Unfortunately, fear and anxiety are all-too-common experiences for individuals with prostate cancer. People with cancer may be afraid that they will pass the disease on to other members of the family. They may be afraid that they will no longer be good family members. They may be afraid that they will not be able to continue working. They may worry more about the treatment than about the cancer itself. They may worry about disfigurement and other body changes. They may worry about *being* afraid.

Often, the emotions experienced by people living with cancer parallel the course of the disease. Feelings are usually most negative during and immediately after the diagnosis, and during any flare-ups that may occur as time goes on. During remissions—periods of time when you genuinely feel good—emotions may be much more positive. Even during remissions, though, anxiety is often a common and very unpleasant part of any type of cancer. And because anxiety can interfere with your ability to deal effectively with any medical problem, it's vital that you learn to cope with this emotion.

People fear cancer more than any other disease. There are many reasons that this is so, including fear of prolonged suffering and fear of deterioration. The reality is that none of these things may come to pass in your case. So the best way to deal with these fears is to obtain as much information as you possibly can. By gaining knowledge and understanding, you will equip yourself to fight and conquer your fears. Just as important, both you and your family can implement successful psychological strategies that will help you deal more effectively with your fears and provide for better adjustment and coping.

WHAT ARE THE SYMPTOMS OF FEAR AND ANXIETY?

What happens when you get extremely anxious? Your body may react physiologically. You may become short of breath, your heart may beat rapidly, you may feel shaky, and you may think, "I've got to get out of here!" You may try to relax, but be unable to do so. You may try to breathe deeply, but find that the breath keeps catching in your throat. You may try to "shake the feeling," but find that you can't. This inability to calm down may become frightening, and may increase your anxiety even more. A vicious cycle may quickly develop. Before long, you may be completely out of control.

Which came first, the anxiety or the symptoms? That's really not important. What's more important is doing whatever is possible to reduce both. And it *is* possible to cope with fear—to regain control of your emotions and improve your day-to-day life.

IS FEAR GOOD OR BAD?

Believe it or not, fear is usually good! Now you're probably saying, "If I'm shaking with fear, how can it be good?" Fear mobilizes you. It tells you to prepare to attack the source of your fear. You react in a way that leads to action. In this regard, fear is similar to stress. It serves a necessary and critical purpose. In a way, it protects you.

Anxiety is bad only when the source of fear becomes overlooked, ignored, or denied, or when the feeling is so excessive that it paralyzes you. In these cases, the threat or danger is allowed to continue, and nothing—or, at least, not enough—is done to control it.

WHAT DETERMINES THE INTENSITY OF OUR REACTIONS?

Fear ranges in intensity from mild to severe. It is impossible to measure how much fear there is in anyone's life. This varies from person to person and from time to time.

What determines how fearful you get? Well, how close is the feared object, person, or event? (Wouldn't you be more afraid if you were getting an injection within the next thirty seconds than you would if you were getting one within thirty days?) How vulnerable are you? (Do you truly hate injections, or are you just tired of feeling like a pincushion?) Finally, how successful are you at defending yourself? (Can you calmly accept the needle, or do you scream a lot?) These are just some of the factors that determine how you handle fear.

Fred, age seventy-one, was afraid to go to sleep at night. He was worried that he'd be awakened in the middle of the night by the need to urinate, which would just remind him of his prostate cancer. If Fred had been emotionally stronger, he still might have experienced some discomfort, but he would not have let this symptom disturb his sleep. However, Fred wasn't a strong person. He allowed the fear to keep him awake, and as he got less and less sleep, he became more and more vulnerable to the very feeling he wanted to avoid!

WHAT IS PANIC?

Although this chapter focuses on fear and anxiety, we really can't discuss these emotions without considering panic. Panic is the most intense form of anxiety—it's what you feel when your anxiety increases beyond the "typical" level. In fact, with panic, the degree of anxiety is so profound that you feel as if you've totally lost control. Research suggests that approximately 5 percent of the general population suffers from panic disorders.

Panic may strike suddenly and without warning. Occasionally, there may not even appear to be a specific trigger. Or the trigger may be perfectly clear, but you may find yourself unable to prevent the panic attack.

Although there are times when anxiety can be beneficial, panic is usually so intense that there are few, if any, benefits to the experience. So let's talk more about panic attacks, and learn what can be done for them.

What Are the Symptoms of Panic Attacks?

The symptoms most common in panic attacks are palpitations, increased heart rate and blood flow, pounding heart, chest pain, sweating, dizziness, shortness of breath, imbalance, disoriented feelings, a feeling of suffocation, rubbery legs, flushing, tingling in different parts of the body, faintness, numbness, nausea, shaking, trembling, a lump in the throat, and light-headedness. Even this sounds frightening! But the list doesn't end there. There are also psychological symptoms, including the feeling of going crazy, the fear of dying, the fear of losing control, a feeling of impending doom, and an urgent desire to escape from the given situation. Wonderful, right?

A number of the physiological symptoms are triggered by sudden bursts of adrenaline, a substance released by the body when you're under stress. This stress response has also been called the "fight or flight" response. (You'll read more about this in Chapter 15.)

Why Is It So Hard to Stop a Panic Attack?

When you are experiencing a panic attack, it may be very difficult to rationally view the situation and realize that there is nothing to be afraid of—or, at least, that your fears may be out of proportion. Rather, you may be unable to think objectively at all, and your emotions may take over. The fear then becomes more and more intense.

The more you feel unable to control panic attacks, the more often they may occur. In part, this happens because you're already out of control, so that it takes less stress to trigger an attack.

There are times when panic attacks are of very short duration. They may last for only a few minutes or so, and then pass. At other times, though, panic attacks may last up to an hour or more. That can be devastating!

The desire to avoid panic attacks may lead to the onset of phobias. Why? Phobias—irrational fears of a situation or object—actually start as avoidance behavior. You may start associating the discomfort of panic attacks with whatever situations you were in at the time that the attacks began. You'll then try to avoid these situations more and more, and finally become phobic in your intense need to avoid the seeming triggers of the attacks.

Fortunately, many of the techniques that are helpful in dealing with fears and anxieties will prevent your emotions from escalating into panic, and will help you deal with panic when it occurs. These strategies include pinpointing possible reasons for your fear and panic, using relaxation techniques to prevent or overcome your panic, and restructuring your thinking. If your feelings of panic continue, though, medication or counseling may be needed. There are also many successful programs designed to help people cope with panic attacks.

HOW CAN YOU COPE WITH FEARS AND ANXIETIES?

Obviously, the more fears you have, the more difficulty you'll experience in making a successful adjustment to your new situation. Recognizing your fears and learning how to deal with them will help you live more happily and more comfortably. How? I was afraid you'd never ask! Let's look at some of the ways in which you can help yourself better cope with your fears. Later in the chapter, we'll look at how you can use some of these strategies—and other strategies as well—to cope with some specific fears that may be troubling you.

Pinpoint the Source of Your Fears

The first step in coping with your fears is to use the pinpointing technique discussed in Chapter 11. Identify and list exactly what you're afraid of and exactly why you are afraid. Then think about what you can do to alleviate your fears. As you begin planning your strategies and gradually putting your plan into operation, you'll feel better and better.

Relax!

Because relaxation is the opposite of tension, the use of relaxation techniques can be very helpful in coping with fears and anxieties. As mentioned earlier in the book, there are many types of relaxation techniques: progressive relaxation, meditation, autogenics, deep breathing, and more. Regardless of what is provoking your fear, learning to relax is an important part of improving emotional well-being. (Detailed information about relaxation techniques can be found in Chapter 19.)

Desensitize Yourself

A great technique used to conquer fear is called *systematic desensitization*. Using this technique, you gradually desensitize yourself—that is, make yourself less vulnerable—to the source of your fear.

Here's how it can work for you. Sit in a comfortable chair and relax. Then create a movie in your mind by imagining whatever it is that makes you afraid. If you get tense, stop imagining it and relax. When you've calmed down, try imagining it again. The more you try to imagine your fear and alternate the "movie" with relaxation techniques, the less it will bother you. Try it! It will give you a great feeling of relaxation and control. There are several library books that provide more information on systematic desensitization. Check them out.

Learn to Cope With Anxious Thoughts

It was stated earlier that anxiety is a vague, uneasy feeling with an unknown source. So how can you cope with anxiety by following the steps listed above? Surely, if you can't pinpoint the source of your fear, you can't follow these specific steps. So what *can* you do? Well, a number of things may work in this case. Try relaxation procedures, discussed earlier in this chapter. Work on changing your thinking to make it more positive and productive. Find somebody you can express your fears to—somebody who will listen to you, talk to you, and try to help you deal with your fears. Even if you can't pinpoint a specific fear, these techniques will greatly help you to cope with general anxiety.

Learn More About Prostate Cancer

Things that are unknown are often things that are feared. And, unfortunately, there is still a lot unknown about cancer. However, the more people you speak to, the more questions you ask, and the more information you obtain, the fewer "unknowns" there will be. This will help to eliminate many of your fears, or at least reduce them to the point at which they're more manageable.

LET'S TALK ABOUT SPECIFICS

When you were first diagnosed, many fearful questions focusing on life probably came to mind. "What will the future be like? What will become of me? Will I die?" These are all typical questions of people who are diagnosed with *any* chronic medical problem, not just prostate cancer. But in the case of cancer, it is particularly common—although usually incorrect—to feel that death may not be far behind.

As time has gone by, in all probability some of these questions have been answered, and you have started to adjust to having cancer. But once these initial fears are reduced, new fears usually focus on more specific questions. In other words, you then focus on the fear of death, the fear of pain, and other possible events and experiences. All of these fears are normal and understandable, and should be expected. But however normal they may be, they can become extremely harmful if you fail to cope with them effectively.

In the previous pages, we looked at some general coping strategies. But you're probably most interested in seeing how these and other strategies can help you better deal with the specific fears that you're struggling with right now. Let's discuss some of these fears and see what methods of coping may help.

Fear of Dying

It's certainly understandable to be afraid of dying. Most people are. And even if the prognosis for your cancer is good, you can be sure that your fears of death will be more prevalent and stronger than they were before the diagnosis.

One problem you may experience in coping with your fear of dying is the fact that you may feel reluctant or unable to discuss it with anybody. It is often very difficult to talk about this fear, especially with people who are close to you. They are usually too quick to tell you not to worry! In addition, you may not always find medical professionals as supportive and understanding as you would like them to be.

When might you be most afraid of dying? It's hard to predict. Certainly, any time you're preparing for a medical exam or test, you will be most vulnerable to this fear. But many people with prostate cancer report that, every now and then, these thoughts fill their minds for no apparent reason.

We've already discussed how fear can sometimes serve a purpose. But being afraid of dying is not going to help you feel better or live longer. If anything, it's going to make you feel worse! So how can you attack this fear? Talk to the people you trust. If necessary, talk to counselors or therapists, who are well equipped to alleviate your fears. Speak to your doctor, if he or she is a compassionate, supportive person. Consider turning to your place of worship, where a religious adviser may be able to help you deal with this fear. Few people have to face the idea of dying alone.

Finally, remember the facts. Remember that medicine is constantly exploring new and improved treatments. So think positively. Many people with prostate cancer live long, comfortable lives. Do you see how you must work on your thinking? If negative thoughts make you more afraid, then positive thoughts . . . !

Fear of Pain

Nobody likes pain. And because pain may may be a problem in advanced prostate cancer, you may be fearful of it. Each little twinge of pain may make you afraid—afraid that your condition is not responding to treatment or that additional problems may develop. And even when you're not in pain, you may fear that it's still to come.

What can you do about this fear? Try to accept the fact that some pain may occur from time to time, but that medication can reduce its intensity, as well as its frequency. Realize that each pain "cycle" will eventually stop, or at least ease up. The pain won't last forever.

Fear of Going to the Doctor

It's not uncommon for people with prostate cancer to become more and more fearful of follow-up medical visits—both visits to doctors' offices and visits to the hospital. They're afraid of what they are going to find out. In fact, in some cases, this fear is so overwhelming that they don't go to the doctor when they should. It's not uncommon for individuals to wait weeks or even months before finally making an appointment. Sometimes they wait as long as years!

As you now know, this is definitely unwise. So make—and keep—your appointments. You're trying to do the best you can with prostate cancer, right? So if there's anything that needs taking care of, you want to find out so that you can take care of it! That doesn't mean you're going to love all of your doctor's visits! But you do want to make the best of them.

Fear of "What Next?"

What will happen next? You can't be sure. Will the cancer spread? Will you develop any side effects from your treatment? Will you develop new symptoms?

Everyone wonders what the future has in store. But because of the unpleasantness of what you're experiencing, you may be *afraid* of the future, rather than merely curious. What can you do? Unless you own a crystal ball, you can't foresee what will happen. So take life one day at a time. What will be, will be. (What a great name for a song!) Just tell yourself that you'll handle any problems as they occur. Keep doing what you have to in order to take care of yourself. That's all you can do, anyway.

Fear of Test Results

Playing the waiting game is one of the most fear-provoking aspects of living with cancer. It can be nerve-wracking to wait for results and wonder what the implications of those results may be. And it sometimes seems as if medical professionals are not aware of the impact of waiting. Often, they take their own sweet time in getting back to you with results. Meanwhile, you feel like you've died a thousand deaths.

What can you do? Focus on your daily activities. Try to keep as busy as you possibly—and realistically—can. This may not totally eliminate these fears from your mind, but it can help the time pass a little more quickly.

Fear of Treatment

Regardless of which treatment your doctor prescribes, there may be frightening things about it—things that may upset you.

Surgery, for instance, may be thought of as deforming, and can bring with it the fear of lost sexual or urinary function. As we've mentioned, advances in surgical technique have decreased the likelihood of either of these problems occurring. But this doesn't mean that you won't fear them, just the same. To deal with this fear, you'll want to work with physicians who you know are board-certified, well trained, and experienced in the field of prostate cancer.

As part of your fear of having surgery, you may fear the loss of parts of your body. You may have never thought about your prostate gland before. You may never have thought about the purpose it served. However, you might now be upset by the fact that after surgery, the prostate may no longer be there. Wouldn't it be better to focus on the anticipated benefits of the surgery? What's more important, after all?

Any fear you have of radiation can be either rational or irrational. It is certainly understandable to be afraid of radiation, since it is such a powerful treatment. However, many fears of radiation are irrational. Deal with these fears—and *all* of your fears regarding treatment of any kind—by asking the questions you need answered beforehand. Be as informed as you can be. Speak to other people who have experienced the treatment. Make sure you understand the purpose of the treatment, the potential for success, and the fact that there are often ways to minimize side effects. By anticipating what may happen, you'll be in much better shape to deal with the possible consequences.

Fear of Recurrence

Even if your cancer treatments are considered to be successful, you still may have fears—fears of a recurrence of cancer. Of course, your doctors will tell you that you have to take care of yourself, and that you must report anything that they should be aware of. This is certainly important. But it is also important not to become so obsessed with self-monitoring that you become cancerphobic! Discuss this with your doctor. Obtain realistic guidelines regarding what you should watch for and what you should disregard. Find out when you should contact your doctor and when you should let things go.

One of the problems with fear of recurrence is that, in many cases, you may have more trouble dealing with a recurrence than you did with your initial bout with cancer. Why? Because once progress has been made, there's a tendency to feel that everything was just a bad dream—a bad dream that's now over. A recurrence may rudely open your eyes once again. In addition, you may be both physically and psychologically weaker at this point, and feel less able to mobilize your defenses.

Don't let these feelings overwhelm you. Speak to people who have been through it. Speak to professionals who are equipped to help you deal with these fears. And remember that whatever occurs, you will be able to cope with it, one day at a time.

Fear of the Reactions of Others

Are you afraid that other people will shy away from you because you have cancer? Because cancer creates such discomfort in society in general, you may be concerned that you will lose friends. You may even fear losing your spouse and other loved ones.

Unfortunately, some people can be cold and unfeeling. They may be put off by the fact that you can no longer keep up with them. But who needs those kinds of friends, anyway? Other friends will accept you under any circumstances. Enjoy them.

Naturally, you should aim to stay involved with family and friends. But be realistic. Remember that a change in a social relationship can occur for any reason, not just because of prostate cancer! And since you can't change the way some people feel, try not to be too concerned with their reactions. Instead, be more attentive to your own needs and feelings.

Of course, if you feel that an important relationship is in jeopardy, you should try to figure out why this might be and to see what you can do to help. And if you feel that people are shying away from you, you should discuss this with them. Try to find out what they are afraid of. Maybe you'll be able to help them. Get counseling, if need be. But remember that you can only do so much. If all your efforts don't work, even though the outcome may upset you, at least you'll know that you did your best.

Finally, if you have been troubled by the reactions of others, you may find it helpful to get involved in a support group. You know that the people in these groups will not shy away from you or abandon you. Why? Because they're going through the same kinds of things that you are! And because of their experiences, participants may even be able to give you tips on dealing with family and friends. (For more information on dealing with others, see Chapters 26–30.)

Fear of Overdoing or Underdoing

You may not know how much you should be doing. You may be afraid of doing too much, but you may feel guilty about doing too little! How can you conquer this fear? Get advice from experts. You'll need professional guidance to come up with the best "mix" of rest and exercise. And you'll need to know which, if any, activities may be too strenuous for you.

Of course, even your doctor may not have specific answers for you. You may be told that the answers will become apparent only through trial-and-error. Experience is the best teacher.

So what should you do? Pace yourself. Change your level of activity gradually. Then tell yourself that, as with so many other fears, you're doing the best you can.

Fear of Dependence

It is very common for individuals with cancer to be fearful of becoming dependent on others. You may fear that you'll lose your independence, as well as your ability to help yourself. And you may fear that as you lose control of your life, the cancer will take control.

You can deal with this fear by concentrating on doing the things that you still can do. Graciously accept the help you may have to take from others, but don't view this new relationship as a dependency. Instead, focus on the benefits you're receiving from your increased interaction with family, friends, and professionals!

Fear of Employment Problems

Like many people with prostate cancer, you may be concerned about the effect your condition will have on your job. You may want to work, but fear that you won't be able to. Your employer may be understanding at first, but you may worry about how long his tolerance will continue. And, of course, because of your medical problems, your need for money will be greater! So if you can't work, the pressure may be tremendous.

What can you do? Talk to people who have been in the same situation, and see what they did. Speak to experts who can advise you on financial matters. Evaluate your vocational skills, and make sure you're equipped to do a job that you can physically handle. And remember that you'll work it out. When was the last time you read of someone being thrown out on the street, penniless, because of prostate cancer?

Fear of Fear

This section could have been called "Fear of Anxiety" or "Fear of Panic Attacks," or any of a number of other things. What they all describe, though, is the response that many people have to bouts of fear and anxiety. Because these emotions are so uncomfortable, many people develop a fear of being afraid. This is called a _secondary anxiety reaction,_ meaning that you're not afraid of a specific object, person, or situation as much as you're anxious about being anxious.

What to do? Start by using relaxation techniques. Then tell yourself that you'll work on dealing with any situation or feeling as it occurs, rather than worrying about what might or might not happen. Reread the information in this chapter. And, if necessary, work with a supportive professional who can help you better cope with this problem.

Fear of Not Coping

You may feel that you're barely handling having prostate cancer. You may think that any new problem that comes along will be enough to push you over the edge. And fear of falling apart can easily lead to panic: an out-of-control feeling that can *make* you fall apart.

Get a hold of yourself. Pinpoint those particular things you're having difficulty with, and get help in dealing with them. Don't wait, and don't project a false sense of bravado. If you feel yourself near the edge, get someone to help you steady yourself. Talk your fears over with someone. Once you have shared your feelings and fears, you may see things a little more clearly. You may be able to deal with problems with greater strength, knowing that you're not alone. And once you're back in control, this fear will disappear.

WHAT PROFESSIONAL TREATMENTS ARE AVAILABLE?

We've discussed a number of things you can do to deal with fears and anxieties. Let's review. You'll want to try to pinpoint what may be triggering your fears, and see if you can change, or even eliminate, these triggers. (If you can't pinpoint them at the time you're anxious, at least try to do so when you have calmed down!) You'll want to desensitize yourself to the source of your fears. You'll want to talk your feelings over with others to gain a fresh perspective. You'll want to use relaxation techniques to increase your sense of being in control. You'll want to work on your thinking, to restructure any negative thoughts that may be contributing to, or exacerbating, the anxiety. And you'll want to learn more about your condition so that you can eliminate any fears of the unknown.

In some cases, using these techniques will bring about a sufficient degree of control. However, there may be times when you need additional help. Let's look at the treatments that may be available for you.

Medication

Medication is one possible means of treating intense fears or panic. The medications used are designed to block whatever is biochemically contributing to the onset or exacerbation of panic. However, keep in mind that although medication may be beneficial in dealing with panic attacks, it may be too aggressive a treatment for some of the lesser fears associated with prostate cancer. But if you feel that medication may be the answer for you, be sure to speak to your doctor. (For more information on medications, see Chapter 18.)

Behavior Therapy

Because fear or panic may lead to additional anxieties and phobias, psychological techniques involving behavior therapy may be helpful as part of treatment. For example, techniques such as systematic desensitization, discussed earlier in the chapter, can be very effective in reducing phobias. A qualified therapist should be able to help you better cope with your fears through the use of behavior therapy.

Psychotherapy

Because intense fear or panic may throw you out of control, you may require professional intervention—especially if these attacks have been occurring often. Don't feel "weak" if you decide to consult a professional. After all, your goal is to feel better, right? If you're having difficulty resolving some of these problems yourself, isn't it good to know that there are experts who can help you regain control?

A FEARLESS SUMMARY

Although many different fears have been discussed in this chapter, we have probably not covered all of the ones you have experienced. In addition, the coping suggestions offered certainly do not include all possible ways of dealing with fear. So what should you do?

Anticipate that you will be fearful of certain things from time to time. Some fears will come back, but plan on riding through them rather than succumbing to them. Remember that it's okay to be scared. Not only is it okay, but it's normal. But also remember that the most important thing is to stay on top of these fears so that they don't overwhelm you or render you less able to cope.

You're working on recognizing your fears, right? For some of them, you're modifying your behavior. For others, you're modifying your thinking. Soon you will feel more in control. As this happens, you'll notice that your fears begin to diminish. That doesn't mean that they'll all go away. But as you work on them, they'll at least lessen in intensity, and you'll feel better knowing that you can handle whatever comes along.

Chapter 13

ANGER

Louie, age fifty-three, was fed up. He was tired of tests, tests, and more tests. He was tired of waiting for the results. He was tired of hearing that there was nothing his doctor could do to speed up his treatment. Practically everyone who went near him received an earful of comments you wouldn't write home about! Everyone, from his doctor to his wife, was a victim of this verbal assault. Was Louie angry? You bet your eardrums he was!

In general, people with any chronic medical problem may be angry. Certainly, it is very common to feel intense anger because of cancer. But because anger results in the buildup of physical energy that needs to be released—in other words, in stress—it's important to learn how to cope with this emotion.

Just what is anger? When you have a desire or goal in mind, and something interferes with efforts to reach this goal, this can be very frustrating. A feeling of tension and hostility may result. This is what we refer to as anger.

Anger may be felt towards the cancer itself, or towards religious beliefs, family, friends, or the medical profession. Virtually anybody may be a target of your anger during your experience with prostate cancer.

Anger can sometimes be an outward manifestation of deeper emotional feelings. Helplessness and frustration—feelings that are more difficult to express—may come out in the form of anger.

ARE THERE DIFFERENT TYPES OF ANGER?

In learning to deal with anger, it can be helpful to discuss the three different ways in which anger can be experienced. This will enable you to more easily identify anger when it does occur.

Rage is the expression of violent, uncontrolled anger. If Louie was feeling upset about his prostate cancer, and a friend told him that he wouldn't be so uncomfortable if he didn't get so "worked up" all the time, you can imagine how angry Louie might be. Louie's anger might even lead him to say or do things that would certainly not enhance the prospects of a long-lasting, friendly relationship with this person!

Rage is probably the most intense anger you can experience. It is an outward expression of anger, because there is noticeable evidence of an explosion. Often, rage is a destructive release of intense physical energy that has built up over time.

A second type of anger is *resentment*. This is a feeling of anger that is usually kept inside. What if Louie listened to his friend's well-meaning comments, smiled, and said nothing, but was seething inside? That emotion would be resentment—a growing, smoldering feeling of anger, directed toward a person or an object, but often kept bottled up. Resentment tends to sit uncomfortably within you, and can create even more physiological and psychological damage than can be caused by rage.

The third type of anger is *indignation*. Indignation is considered a more appropriate, positive type of anger, as, unlike resentment, it is released, but in a controlled way. If Louie had responded to his friend's comments by stating that he appreciated the concern, but would prefer no advice at this point—or he might flatten him—this would have been an expression of indignation.

Obviously, these three types of anger can occur in combination and in many different ways. However, understanding the different ways of experiencing anger can help you to identify and cope with it more effectively.

WHAT CAUSES ANGER?

There are, of course, lots of things that can make you angry. You may get angry if you have to wait to see your doctor. You may get angry if you feel that your family is not understanding enough. You may get angry if you feel that the prescribed treatment isn't helping you.

Thoughtless comments from other people can cause anger, as well. For example, "If you drank more fluids, you wouldn't have those problems," is not the kind of comment that will make you feel friendly! If you sense that someone is taking advantage of you, or if you feel forced to do something that you do not want to do, anger may result. If you do not have the ability or confidence to say "no" when friends ask for a favor, this, too, can create feelings of anger—especially if you feel too fatigued to complete even your own tasks!

In addition to the causes of anger mentioned above, there is one more. How about prostate cancer? Aren't you angry about this? Being aware of this is important, because you must be aware of anger before you can deal with it. Unfortunately, resolving your anger won't make the prostate cancer go away. Nor should you say that you'll stop being angry only if your cancer is cured. Neither attitude will help you.

In their anger over having prostate cancer, one of the most common questions that people ask is, "Why me?" This question suggests that what happened shouldn't have happened—that it's unfair, or that someone or something is somehow to blame. Again, it's important to realize that the anger in this case is not helpful—that asking "Why me?" will not benefit you in any way. It's far better to ask yourself what you can do about it now that it *has* happened. And this book is full of things that you can do to help yourself feel better, both physically and mentally, including things you can do to reduce your anger.

Before we finish looking at the causes of anger, it is important to realize that anger exists uniquely in the mind of each angry individual. Anger is a direct result of your thoughts, not of events. The event by itself does not make you angry. Rather, your anger is caused by your interpretation of the event—the way you think or feel about it. This is a very important point, and one that will be discussed in much more detail a little bit later, in the section "How Can You Cope With Anger?" Stay tuned . . .

HOW DOES ANGER AFFECT YOUR BODY?

When you are angry, a number of physiological responses occur. Your breathing becomes more rapid, your blood pressure increases (you may feel like your blood is "boiling"), and your heart may begin to pound. Your face may get "hot," and your muscles may tense. You may also feel stronger when angry. The more intense the anger is, the greater this feeling of power. In fact, you may be able to remember a time when you were so angry that you felt you had superhuman strength.

Anger is a form of energy. The more physical energy that builds up in the body due to anger, the more necessary it becomes to release it. This energy cannot be destroyed. So if it is not released in some constructive manner, it will eventually come out in another, less desirable way.

Imagine that the energy from anger is a stick of dynamite about to explode. If you get rid of it, it may cause some damage when it explodes, but it will not hurt you as much as it would if you swallowed it to keep others from being hurt. Obviously, the ideal solution is to neither throw nor swallow the dynamite, but—are you ready for this?—to defuse it! (More about defusing later in the chapter.)

Usually, extreme anger passes quickly. If, however, the anger lasts for a long period of time, it can have physically damaging effects on the body. You've probably heard about some of the physical problems that can result from holding in anger, such as ulcers, hypertension, and headaches. Well, anger can also exacerbate existing medical problems. It's just not good for your body.

HOW DOES ANGER AFFECT YOUR MIND?

Anger is usually experienced as a very unpleasant feeling. However, this unpleasant feeling may exist along with a more pleasurable feeling of power or strength. Frequently, the unpleasantness of anger is related to its consequences—knowing what you do when you are angry, and not being happy about it. Sometimes, anger may become so extreme that you feel like exploding. You may feel that unless you are able to punch, kick, or hit something—to get rid of the anger in some way—you will lose control. Hopefully, this angry energy can be released without causing damage to another person, to property, or to yourself. If, when you finally calm down, you find that you have done something destructive, you may get angry at yourself all over again. Or you may experience another negative emotion, such as guilt.

IS ANGER GOOD OR BAD?

You may wonder how anger could possibly be good. Certainly, many people feel that nothing constructive can be gained from anger. "Avoid anger at all costs," they say, "because nothing good can come of it." This is true only if you don't deal with anger properly. Anger can, indeed, be dangerous if it's kept inside or released in inappropriate ways.

Remember that stick of dynamite? What an explosive example! If anger is released in destructive ways, it can cause problems in relationships—to say the least! It can also aggravate the medical problems you're already trying to deal with. Does this mean that anger can make your condition worse? Well, what if you're so angry at somebody—your doctor, say, or an overprotective friend—that you don't follow your treatment program, or you do more than you should? "I'll show them," you say. And then you go on to exhaust yourself. In this case, obviously, anger is harmful, but only because you've turned it against yourself.

But anger can also be constructive. How? First, it can give you an indication that something is wrong—something that needs attention. Second, it can motivate you to deal more actively with life's problems.

Anger can give you a feeling of power or strength, of confidence or assertiveness. But don't get me wrong. I'm not saying that you should slam your finger with a hammer or tell someone to punch you in order to get yourself angry enough to solve your problems! What I am saying is that anger can be positive, and, if used correctly, can help you find solutions to real problems.

SOME DIFFERENT REACTIONS TO ANGER

Marty, a fifty-eight-year-old attorney, was having a hard time with his wife. She was trying to show concern for her husband by relieving him of all responsibilities around the house. But, surprisingly, he wanted to help. He felt well enough to continue doing household chores, and he wanted to be treated as normally as possible. *He* wanted to be the one to determine when he would be active. Marty's wife just couldn't see this, and Marty was running out of patience. Let's look at three ways in which this situation might be handled.

The "Just Ignore It" Approach

If you feel overwhelmed by the intensity of your anger and fear that you may completely lose control, you may try to do whatever you can to avoid the experience. This could include pushing any angry thoughts out of your mind, no matter how important the issue is to you.

So rather than making a fuss over household responsibilities, Marty could try to get involved in other activities and ignore the fact that his wife was being condescending. Or he could try to agree with everything that she said. Although this might be upsetting, it would at least be temporarily effective in helping Marty ignore his wife's attitude. In the long run, however, you can see that this would not be the best way in which Marty could deal with his anger.

The "Take Power" Approach

Maybe you enjoy the flow of energy and strength that comes from being angry. You may find that when you're angry, you are best able to assert yourself and get things done.

Marty might know that if he was smothered once too often, he would explode—and he might love the feeling of power that this anger gives him. He might almost look forward to the chance to say, "Honey, if you treat me that way once more, I'll take this vacuum cleaner and ... !" That would wipe the smile off his wife's face!

If you enjoy this feeling, it's possible that you may even provoke situations to make yourself angry. Perhaps you've heard of professional football players or boxers who psych themselves before a confrontation with an opponent. For them, getting angry is the best preparation for a successful performance!

The "Take Action" Approach

It's possible to see anger as a necessary, though unpleasant, part of life. You know that there will be times when you'll be angry, whether you like it or not. But you can choose to deal with both your anger and the situation that's causing it as effectively as possible.

For example, Marty might recognize that he's not happy being angry, but realize that he should speak to his wife so that she can better understand his emotional needs. In this case, even if Marty failed to persuade his wife to let him assume his normal household responsibilities, he would at least have the satisfaction of knowing that he did something about his feelings.

Your own reaction to anger is unique. It may also change from time to time. There may be times when you accept anger and almost value it as a motivator. At other times you may attempt to push this anger away. Marty might enjoy expressing his anger. But if he didn't want to hurt his wife or upset the rest of the family, he might choose to have a calm discussion rather than shattering everyone's eardrums with his explosion.

Of course, the way in which you deal with your emotions now is probably similar to the way in which you've dealt with adversity in the past. If you have always dealt with problems in a generally positive, constructive manner, you will probably deal with any new problems in a positive way. On the other hand, if you have had difficulty in dealing with stress in the past, you may also have difficulty dealing with it now. But remember that you can *learn* to effectively cope with anger, just as Marty did in the third example. Let's learn more about this.

HOW CAN YOU COPE WITH ANGER?

You've already begun to realize that anger can be constructive. Hopefully, the information you've read so far has been encouraging. But what, specifically, can you do to cope with your anger?

Because anger is such a complex emotion, and because so many things can lead to feelings of anger, there are no simple answers. (Sorry about that!) Does that mean that there is nothing that anybody can do about anger? No. There are many things that can be done to reduce your feelings of anger and to handle them more efficiently, comfortably, and safely. First, of course, you'll have to be able to admit that you're angry, and to figure out why you're angry. Once you've pinpointed the source of your anger, you may be able to defuse your anger, or, if that's not possible, to find an acceptable outlet for it. Let's take a look at each of these ways of coping with anger.

Recognize Your Anger

There are two steps involved in recognizing that you're angry: admitting its existence, and identifying its source. Let's discuss these in greater detail.

Step One: Admit That You're Angry

The first step in dealing with anger is to recognize that you're angry in the first place. As simple as this may sound, many people cannot admit being angry. They may try to deny it, or they may rationalize their feelings or behavior using other explanations.

Do you feel that being angry is a sign of weakness? If so, you may not admit that you're angry—perhaps not even to yourself. You may feel that there is no appropriate reason to be angry, and that anger is a childish reaction. But, as with anything else, in order to change something, you have to recognize that it exists.

How can you tell if you're angry? (Yes, there are some people who are not sure.) If you feel very tense (jumping at the sound of the telephone), or if you find yourself reacting with impulsiveness (slamming down the phone when you get a wrong number and storming out of the house) or hostility (cursing at your neighbor for leaving a smidgeon of garbage on your lawn), chances are that you're angry. Don't be afraid to recognize it, as this is the first step in dealing with it.

Step Two: Identify the Source of Your Anger

The second step in dealing with anger is trying to identify its source. Where did the anger come from? What is contributing to it? What events have led to this feeling of anger? Why do you want to break all the furniture?

For one thing, as we mentioned earlier in the chapter, your condition may lead to anger. You may feel anger towards your physician, whether justified or not. You may be angry because you have cancer. You may be angry because you feel so out of control. In some cases, the events leading to an angry reaction may be quite obvious. In other cases, however, it may be hard to pinpoint the cause. At such times, try to probe deeply to find the source of the problem.

Take the case of Stuart, a fifty-seven-year-old salesman. Stuart was awakened one bright, cheerful morning to the singing of birds outside his bedroom. Instead of feeling happy and carefree, though, he felt angry. He had just awakened, but he felt angry. At first, he couldn't figure out why he felt angry on such a beautiful day. But finally, after giving the matter a lot of thought, he realized that because it was sunny and bright out, his detested cousins were going to come from out of town to visit, and he would feel obligated to entertain them—something that he did not wish to do.

So, at this point, it's necessary to explain to yourself why you're angry. Why is this step important? Because you want to decide whether or not the anger you're feeling is realistic. If necessary, write down what you think is making you angry. Be honest when writing down your thoughts, regardless of how violent or profane they may be! Rich, colorful language can be helpful in getting your feelings out, and will ultimately allow you to control your anger. Try to look at these thoughts objectively, the way someone else might look at them. If, like Stuart, you recognize that your reasons are not rational, this alone may help you to deal with your feelings. If, on the other hand, you can objectively say that your feelings of anger are rational, your next step step will be to decide how you can properly cope with them.

How *can* you cope with them properly? You've already begun! By working through these steps, you have received information that will be very helpful in your efforts to deal with your anger. Now, depending on the situation, you can either defuse your anger or find an outlet for it. Read on to see how each of these choices can work for you!

Defuse Your Anger

In the past, it was falsely believed that there were only two possible ways to deal with anger: to keep it inside, or to let it out. But what about a third possibility? Remember when we talked about defusing that stick of dynamite? Your anger is a result of the way you think! In your mind, you're interpreting events in a way that makes you angry. So if you can change the way you interpret events and reorganize your thinking patterns, you can actually stop creating the anger that you feel. Is this really possible? Well, ask yourself this question: If something happened that made you angry, would everybody in the world be angry because of it? No. The reason you'd be angry is that this would be the way *you* would think about, or interpret, the event. Other people might not be angry because they might not interpret the event in the same way. Let's look at some of the ways you can defuse your anger *before* it becomes a problem.

Watch Mental Movies

When you become angry, you frequently have all kinds of pictures in your head—images of what's making you angry and of how you'd like to deal with your feelings. These "mental movies" can be a helpful means of defusing your anger.

For example, imagine that you are very, very tired. Your friend calls to tell you that his car has broken down. Could you please pick him up? When you tell him that you are too tired to go out, he says something about how he can never depend on you for anything. This is a friend? You are irate. At that moment, ask your friend to hold on, close your eyes, and imagine all the abusive things that you'd like to say to him. Then imagine the shocked expression on his face. After using this mental imagery, you'll probably be able to complete the phone call without destroying a friendship. You may even smile or laugh as you think about the scenes that are playing through your mind. (More about imagery in Chapter 19.)

Norton was quite fed up with his son, Pesty Pete. Whenever he asked for Pete's help around the house, the child's answers were fresh and abusive. Just before Norton was about to give his son a haircut with a meat cleaver, he remembered the mental movie technique. Norton then imagined himself strangling his son—his eyeballs popping, and gurgling sounds coming from his throat. This helped to rid Norton of the intense, angry feelings that were making him crazy, and allowed him to deal with Pete more constructively. Norton was lucky in that he was eventually able to enlist his son's help by giving him additional privileges. But keep in mind that even if Norton had simply realized that there was no way in which he could change his son's behavior, that very realization would have been constructive. How? It would have allowed Norton to move on and seek solutions that didn't require his son's help. (For more information on dealing with others, see Chapters 26 through 30.)

Picture a Big Red Stop Sign

Another technique that can help you to control anger is referred to as *thought stopping*. Remember: It is the *thoughts* in your mind that are making you angry—the thoughts you have when you interpret an event. When you find that angry thoughts have come into your head, picture a big red stop sign. Seeing that picture in your mind will serve as a momentary distraction. Then concentrate on something you enjoy. This can be a peaceful, relaxing scene, a type of food that you like, an activity that you enjoy, or a favorite movie or television program. Whatever you choose, you will divert your thinking and give yourself a chance to dissipate your anger. You could also participate in a pleasant activity— reading a book, taking a walk, or watching a ball game, for instance. Any of these activities should help to defuse your anger.

Change Your Requirements

At times, you may have specific requirements—particular ways in which you want certain things to occur. Then, when your requirements are not met, you may feel angry. Trying to modify your requirements can help you to cope with your anger.

Let's say that you're not feeling well and you decide to call your doctor. The answering service tells you that he is not in the office and that you should get a return call within a half hour. After forty-five minutes, the doctor has not yet returned your call, and you are fuming. Why? Because your requirement of having your call returned within thirty minutes was not met.

What to do? Revise your requirement. Tell yourself that you would have liked a call within thirty minutes, but that your doctor may be tied up on another case, or in transit, or unable to get to a phone. You'll be satisfied if you get a call at his earliest convenience. By modifying the requirement, you can feel less angry.

Another way to benefit from this technique is to write your require-ments down on paper. Then try to write down new, more flexible desires. This may help you to see your requirements in a new, more objective light.

Put Yourself in the Other Person's Shoes

One of the best ways of dealing with anger towards somebody else is to try to understand exactly what that person is feeling—what the person wants, or why the person is saying what he or she is saying. This will make you more aware of the reason for the behavior, and will also help you deal with it more constructively. Perhaps just as important, this technique can help you understand how that other person will feel if he or she is the target of an abusive release of anger.

Joe always got angry when his wife insisted that he go shopping with her, especially when he was so tired that he couldn't even enjoy watching a football game on TV. Because his anger was exhausting him even further, Joe knew that he had to find a better way of dealing with it. Rather than exploding, Joe imagined how his wife was feeling—how disappointed she was because, after all, she simply wanted to spend more time with him and to enjoy his company while shopping. Joe's new understanding allowed him to defuse his anger and to more effectively explain why he simply couldn't accompany his wife on her errands.

Let Your Anger Out

We have now discussed a number of ways in which you can control your thinking and improve your ability to interpret events in ways that will prevent anger from growing. But these techniques might not always be successful. What if there are times when you *remain* angry? What can be done to deal with anger constructively when it can't be defused? Fortunately, there are two possibilities. Let's see what they are.

Talk, Don't Bite

Obviously, it is much more desirable to have a constructive discussion over an issue than it is to have an angry exchange of heated words that accomplish nothing. In most cases, anger arises when you have a conflict or problem with another person. For this reason, it can be very helpful to learn how to get your points across constructively so that you can negotiate a solution. Remember that a heated argument—fighting fire with fire—is not the answer. Instead, you want to fight the fire by dousing it—by reducing the heatedness of the argument.

How can this be done? Try complimenting the person or looking for the positive things in what that person is saying to you. Yes, do this even though you're angry. This will work in two ways. First, it will probably surprise the person. And how will this help? Well, part of what fuels the fire of anger is your anticipation of the other person's anger. So by catching that person off guard, and thereby preventing him or her from reacting with anger, you will reduce this fuel. Second, by focusing on words or thoughts that are more constructive, you will calm yourself, rather than letting your anger grow. And once you're calm, you'll be able to quietly state your feelings.

Let's take the earlier example in which you became upset by your friend's demands to pick him up. Instead of blowing up at him and telling him how inconsiderate he is, tell your friend that he was right to call you—that you're glad he thought of you. But then let him know that as much as you would like to do this favor for him, you don't have the strength to even get dressed. Regardless of what he says, keep looking for a positive way to respond, and continue to calmly indicate that you don't feel well. Eventually, you'll get your point across. Although he may not be too happy about it—he may even get angry—you will have resolved a problem in a constructive way, with much less anger.

Find a Physical Release for Your Anger

In general, one of the best outlets for releasing angry energy is physical activity. But what if—because of prostate cancer, or your age, or any other reason—this outlet is not as available as you'd like? Fortunately, there are solutions.

Some people find that physical energy from anger can be released by *watching* things! For example, by watching a sporting event, you won't be able to release energy through participation in the sport, but you may be able to release your anger by "getting into" the activities you're viewing. Or you might try watching a particularly violent or emotionally draining movie. You may become so totally absorbed that your built-up energy is released through worry, fear, or excitement. A book that allows you to identify with the characters can be beneficial as well—especially if the characters themselves release anger.

Believe it or not, a common and very effective outlet for anger is crying. I'm sure you've heard of the therapeutic effects of a good cry. However, this technique is not for everyone. For instance, you may not think that it's "manly" to cry—although you might be amazed by the number of men who unashamedly let their tears flow. But if your anger has built up to the point of uncontrollable crying, this will be a great way to let it out. (Of course, you may scare the daylights out of your family. But just tell them you read about it here!)

Some people like to count to ten when angry. This may distract you from what is making you angry, and give you a chance to calm down and think about it more constructively. Try counting out loud, and expressing your feelings through facial expressions and tone of voice. Count to a thousand, if necessary!

AN ANGER-LESS SUMMARY

As you learn to cope with your anger, it's important to remember that events alone do not make you angry. It is your thinking—your interpretation of these events—that leads to anger. And since it is your thinking that makes you angry, you are responsible for feeling this way. Therefore, you can be just as responsible for changing your thinking to help yourself cope with anger—or, at least, to reduce it to a more manageable level.

The best way to handle anger is to be in control so that it doesn't build up in the first place—to restructure your thinking so that your emotions don't get out of hand. But if anger does build, remember that when anger is channeled and used constructively, it can have its benefits. And when this isn't possible, you can defuse or release your anger in a way that harms neither you nor anybody else.

Chapter 14

GUILT

Have you ever felt guilty? Many individuals with prostate cancer say that they have. In fact, guilt is a common emotion not only of people with cancer, but of their family members, as well.

Certainly, guilt is a very unpleasant feeling. Take the case of Abe, a fifty-five-year-old father of three. Before Abe's prostate cancer diagnosis, one of his favorite activities was playing tennis with his wife. Then his doctor suggested that he try more sedentary activities for a while. As a result, Abe felt guilty because he was no longer engaging in an activity that he knew made his wife happy. In fact, Abe felt that he was a bad husband. Was this guilt hard to cope with? You bet! But Abe didn't *have* to be a victim of guilt. Let's first take a look at what leads to guilty feelings, and then look at some ways in which you can reduce your feelings of guilt. After all, you want to do everything possible to make yourself feel better, and it's hard to feel good when you're feeling guilty!

WHAT ARE THE TWO COMPONENTS OF GUILT?

Feelings of guilt usually have two components. The first of these is the sense of "wrongdoing"—the feeling that you have either done something wrong, or that you haven't done something that you should have done. The second component is the feeling of "badness" that results from this self-blame. And it's this second component that's the true culprit! When you feel bad about doing something wrong, this is normal and understandable. But when you start telling yourself that you *are* bad, guilt follows.

WHAT CAUSES GUILT?

There are a lot of things you might feel guilty about, even though, in all likelihood, there's no validity to any of them. For example, maybe you're concerned about what you did to contribute to the development of your cancer. You may feel guilty that you didn't take care of yourself properly—that, perhaps, you waited too long before having a symptom of the disorder attended to—and that if it weren't for certain actions (or lack of actions) on your part, you would not be in this situation. Or guilt may develop simply because you are not able to find any rational reason for the disease. Therefore, you blame yourself.

You may also feel guilty because of feelings that you're complicating things for your family. You may worry that you're not going to be the kind of family member you'd like to be or that you're expected to be. You may feel guilty about letting yourself down or about letting others down, whether they be family, friends, or colleagues.

You may also feel guilty because of feelings you have towards other people—feelings of resentment, perhaps, or jealousy—because they don't have cancer.

Perhaps people have told you that your feelings of guilt have no rational basis—that you're not at fault. Unfortunately, this may not eliminate the guilt. Why? Because your feelings of guilt may have nothing to do with what others say or think. Remember: Your guilt comes from your own feeling that you are a bad person.

Obviously, guilt can be a destructive emotion. It can drain you physically and emotionally, and can undermine your efforts to cope successfully with prostate cancer. Fortunately, there's plenty you can do to improve your outlook. In the remainder of the chapter, we'll look at the various techniques you can use to cope with guilt.

HOW CAN YOU COPE WITH GUILT?

Regardless of the cause of your guilt—and regardless of whether this is a new or long-standing problem for you—there are a number of strategies that can help you reduce or eliminate this unpleasant and harmful emotion. Let's take a look at a few of the best ways of coping with guilt.

Find the Source of Your Guilt

In order to successfully cope with guilt, you must first focus on what led to the guilty feelings. Sometimes, just by pinpointing the source of this emotion, you can greatly reduce the feeling, or even eliminate it.

First, ask yourself if you have actually done something wrong. If you feel you have, ask yourself if the behavior that you're blaming yourself for was really that terrible. In Abe's case, as discussed earlier, Abe felt guilty because of his prostate cancer. Did that make sense? Did he make it happen? Of course not. Identify the cause of your guilt and examine the wrongdoing you feel you committed. You will probably find that you either are not responsible for the wrong action, or that the action was really not terrible enough to justify the feeling of badness that led to your guilt!

Sometimes, people feel guilty about thoughts or desires, rather than specific actions or behaviors. Recognize the difference between feeling guilty over an action and feeling guilty over a thought. Then, once you've identified the thought that's making you feel like a bad person, change that thought. Learn to talk to yourself in a positive way. Look at the thoughts objectively and constructively in order to reduce your guilt.

Mark, a sixty-four-year-old plumber, felt angry about his prostate cancer, and also was extremely lonely because no one seemed to understand what he was going through. It occurred to Mark that he would feel less isolated if his neighbor and best friend, Jim, also had prostate cancer. This thought, of course, caused Mark great feelings of guilt. How could he possibly wish prostate cancer on his best friend? Gradually, though, Mark came to realize that he did not really want his friend to have cancer; he was simply trying to deal with his own loneliness and anger. By understanding this, and by using strategies to better handle his emotions, Mark not only eliminated his guilt but also improved his whole outlook.

But what if you feel guilty and you simply can't remember what you were thinking or doing that made you feel this way? How can you use all the great thought-changing ideas we're going to talk about if you can't identify the thoughts you want to change? Good question! In order to pinpoint these "target" thoughts or behaviors, you might want to keep a brief written log of feelings or activities that may be causing your guilt. Once you have written these things down, you can begin to determine the root of the problem, and then think about what changes might improve the situation.

Benny, age fifty-nine, had been feeling increasingly guilty, but didn't really know why. By keeping a log, he noticed that, besides complaining of fatigue all of time, he had been arriving at work late on a regular basis. He wasn't aware of how frequently he had been late—and he had always been so proud of his punctuality! The log helped him to see that he needed to change his morning routine in order to be more punctual. As he worked on this problem, his guilt lessened.

Talk It Over

It's very important to discuss how you feel about your condition with others who may be affected by it. Share your concerns, and try to figure out solutions to any problems that exist.

Mike, age fifty-nine, had enjoyed a very active social life before being diagnosed with prostate cancer. In addition to going out on weekends, he and his wife would play golf with friends or participate in other social activities at least two or three evenings a week. Now, because of the way prostate cancer was affecting him, Mike had to temporarily restrict his activities. He just couldn't go out as frequently as he used to. Sometimes, he couldn't go out even once during an entire week! Naturally, Mike did not feel happy about his new limitations. In addition, he felt extremely guilty about holding his wife back. He felt that she couldn't have a good time because of him.

Fortunately, Mike had the good sense to sit down with his wife and discuss the situation. Together, they decided that until Mike regained some of his strength, either he would drive his wife's golf cart and accompany her when she played, or he would rest at home while she played with friends. To end their discussion on a positive note, Mike and his wife chose which golf course they would play on as soon as Mike felt up to participating in the game. Mike felt better, knowing that his limitations would not prevent his wife from enjoying her favorite sport. Mike now also had something specific to look forward to—a shared game on a beautiful course.

Turn Your Thoughts Around

Is there anything you can do about the negative thoughts that lead to guilt—those thoughts that make you feel that you're a bad person? One helpful thing you can do is to try to restructure your thinking to make it more positive and guilt-free.

For example, let's say that you feel guilty because you believe that you're not being a good father. Ask yourself if you've ever done *anything* that a good father might do. Just about every dad can come up with something! This type of thinking will begin to eliminate your "bad father blues." The idea is to turn your mind's negative thoughts into reasonable, positive ones. This way, the feeling of guilt will not take a stranglehold!

Evaluate Your Goals

Because of his prostate cancer, Carl, age sixty-one, was not able to work as hard has he had before his diagnosis. He therefore earned less money, and couldn't provide all of the luxuries he and his family would have enjoyed. Feeling guilty, Carl tried to work harder to increase his earnings, which in turn made him feel worse physically. Obviously, Carl was not coping well with his guilt. Instead, he was allowing it to affect his health.

Do you, like Carl, see a difference between the way you *are* doing something and the way you *think* you should be doing it? If so, you are probably feeling guilty! How can you work this out? Major union-management problems might seem easier to solve! Can you work harder or do more? If you can, and it's appropriate for you to do so, then you've solved your problem. If not, though, try examining your day-to-day goals for working and living. Ask yourself if these goals are practical, considering what you can and cannot do because of your prostate cancer.

When evaluating your goals, you may find that among the most common causes of guilt are thoughts containing the word "should." "Should" is a dirty word! Carl thought that he "should" have been able to work harder and earn more money. Other "should" thoughts might include, "I should have been able to finish painting that room today," and "I really should be changing the oil in my car myself, instead of taking it to the service station." These "should" thoughts imply that you must be just about perfect and right on top of everything. Naturally, you will become upset whenever you fall short of your "should." But should you blame yourself when "should" thoughts establish goals that that are unrealistic—goals that you may not be able to fulfill? Obviously, you shouldn't!

Now that I've explained what you shouldn't do, what exactly should you do? In order to feel better and reduce your feelings of guilt, reword your thoughts to eliminate the word "should." Use less demanding words instead. Say, "It would be nice if I could finish that task today, but I can't," rather than, "I should finish that task today." If you have trouble changing the wording of your "should" thoughts, try asking yourself, "Why should I?" or "Who says I should?" or "Where is it written that I should?" This may help you decide whether you are setting up impossible requirements for yourself. It can also help you to reduce your feelings of guilt.

Let's say, for example, that you are thinking of having a party because all of your friends have invited you to get-togethers. Ask yourself *why* you should. Is it because the "Party Rulebook" tells you that if you don't have a party, your friendship license will be revoked? Is it because if you don't have a party, your friends—some friends!—won't invite you to their homes anymore? As you think about the realistic answers to these questions, it will be easier to realize that you don't *have* to have a party. Although it would be nice, it would be more sensible to wait until you're feeling better.

Another way you can eliminate guilt feelings over "should" thoughts is to take more pride in what you can do, rather than focusing on things you feel you should do, but that you might not be up to at this time. Although most people hate hearing that "things could be worse," this is quite true. There are people who can't do anything at all. If you concentrate on the things you can do, and dwell less on what you can't, your feelings of guilt will diminish, and you'll feel a lot better. Changing the emphasis in your thinking will also help you lessen the perceived gap between what is and what you feel "should" be—which is what led to these guilty feelings in the first place.

Escape From Escape Behavior

Sometimes, people who feel guilt—and have failed to cope with this destructive emotion—act in negative ways to hide from their feelings. There may be a tendency to indulge in "escape" behaviors, such as drinking or excessive sleeping—behavior that does not deal with problems head-on, but, instead, attempts to push them away.

As you may have already guessed, the first step towards improvement is to look past the escape behavior and identify what is causing the guilt. Then consider what can be done to rectify the problem. At the same time, try to eliminate the escape behavior, recognizing that this activity is not improving your situation in any way. If you have difficulty eliminating this behavior by yourself—or, for that matter, in identifying the root of the problem—by all means consider working with a supportive professional. You're worth it!

It is possible, of course, that there is no clear-cut way to eliminate the situation or feelings that have led to your guilt. But don't give up. Instead, look for partial solutions. These may not be as desirable as complete solutions, but they can still help to reduce your guilt and make you feel better about yourself.

A FINAL GUILTLESS THOUGHT

Guilt is a very destructive emotion—one that can interfere with your success in coping with prostate cancer by lowering your self-image and exhausting your emotional resources. By becoming aware of how guilt develops, by pinpointing the source of your guilt, and by changing your thinking to be more positive and realistic, you should be able to decrease or eliminate this feeling, and, instead, use your energy to successfully cope with your condition.

Chapter 15

STRESS

Stress. Stress! Every time you turn around, you read or hear about stress. What exactly is stress? Stress is a response that occurs in your body. Stress is a form of energy—a normal reaction to the demands of everyday life. It helps you mobilize your strength to deal with different events and circumstances.

Many things occur each day that require you to adapt. These are the *stressors*. All the changes that take place in your body when something (the stressor) provokes you are known as the *stress response*.

By now, everyone knows that stress can play a role in causing or exacerbating virtually every medical problem. And prostate cancer is no exception. In fact, any cancer experience both causes stress and can be affected by stress.

So chances are you've been feeling pretty stressed lately, and you'd be a lot happier if you could lower your level of stress. Let's learn more about stress—about what causes it, how it can affect you, and, most important, how you can learn to cope with it.

WHAT ARE THE SYMPTOMS OF STRESS?

Your body will tell you when the stress you're experiencing is excessive. What might you feel? Physically, excessive stress can manifest itself as sweaty palms, heart palpitations, tightness of the throat, nausea, diarrhea, and headaches—among other delightful feelings. Emotionally, fatigue, depression, anxiety, anger, frustration, or simply a vague uneasiness are just a few of the possible symptoms of stress. So you can see that as long as you tune into your body and mind, you'll know when you can benefit from some stress-reduction techniques.

HOW DOES STRESS AFFECT YOU?

Now you know some of the many possible symptoms of stress. But the effects of stress—like the effects of depression, discussed in Chapter

11—are not isolated problems. Instead, they are part of a complex response that can affect both your body and your emotions. Let's examine this in more detail.

How Stress Affects Your Body

Stress is a natural survival response. It occurs within the body any time you feel threatened by thoughts or external stressors.

Stress can manifest itself in many ways. When you experience a stressful situation, the circulatory system speeds up, and blood is pushed rapidly towards different parts of the body—particularly those organs and systems necessary to protect you—raising your blood pressure. Because the blood supply has been diverted, the supply to the digestive system is usually reduced, making the the process of digestion slower and less effective. Stress also constricts the blood vessels, increases heart rate, and produces other physiological manifestations. (And it does all these things instantaneously!)

What else can occur? You may tremble or perspire. Your face may flush. You may feel a surge of adrenaline flowing through your body. Your mouth may become dry, and you may feel nauseous. Your breathing may become more rapid and shallow. Your heart may begin to pound. Your muscles may become tight, leading to headaches or cramps. Sounds wonderful, doesn't it?

So, when you experience stress, your body physiologically prepares itself to counter a threat to its survival. Why? Well, perhaps you've heard of the "fight or flight" response. You see, when an animal feels threatened, it prepares to either fight or run away. You will not see an animal standing there, scratching his head, and thinking about how he might best handle the situation. Even though you have the ability to think and reason, you also experience the "fight or flight" response, which causes many different hormones to be secreted, and tenses your muscles in preparation for battle. If the response does involve physical action—fight or flight—the hormones are utilized as they are supposed to be, and the muscles are exercised, with energy being appropriately released. However, if there is no physical exertion—if you think instead of taking action—the energy that was mobilized may not be released in the way expected. This may explain why after a period of stress during which you haven't taken any action, you feel exhausted just the same.

When does stress lead to physical problems? When you can't respond to stress in a way that eliminates it, the stress continues unabated—and so do its symptoms. An inability to do anything to relieve the stress may cause even more stress, creating a vicious cycle. And this can take its toll on your body. In fact, many researchers believe that prolonged stress puts such a strain on your body that your immune system may break down, making your body vulnerable to a number of illnesses, including cancer.

How Stress Affects Your Mind

Your emotional response to stress may not be as visible as your physical response. You may start worrying, get upset, and fear the next "event." Your attention span may be reduced, and you may be less able to concentrate on the task at hand. You may have trouble learning something new. You may be afraid to do things. You may withdraw or feel nervous. You may lose confidence in yourself.

As you become nervous and upset, you may become more aware of any unpleasant physical responses you're experiencing, and this may make you feel even more stressed. For example, if you have responded to stress with shallow, rapid breathing or heart palpitations, your awareness of these physical responses may lead to feelings of panic. Most people respond to stress both physically and emotionally, although it is possible to respond in only one way. Don't you have your own "typical" reaction? Maybe you become too jittery and unfocused to concentrate on your job. Maybe you feel physically ill, with extreme intestinal discomfort or a throbbing headache. However you feel, it's clear that it's important to learn strategies that will enable you to deal effectively with stress.

THREE REACTIONS TO STRESS

We've just discussed how your body and mind respond to stress. But we also want to look at a third type of response—the way that you *choose* to deal with stress.

When a stressful stimulus occurs, you will most likely react in one of three ways. You might not respond at all, and either "go with the flow" or become unable to function. You might respond immediately and impulsively without giving thought to whether a better response might be possible. Or you might respond to stressors in a well-planned, organized, and effective manner. If so, you may not even need this chapter! But if not, read on!

IS STRESS GOOD OR BAD?

By now, you've probably figured out that stress can be either good or bad. It is good when it gives you extra energy to do the things that you need to do during stressful times. In fact, a certain amount of stress is normal and necessary. Stress helps you to "get your act together," and prepares you to handle your life in the best possible way. But when stress is left unchecked, it can be highly destructive, draining all of your energy and possibly worsening any physical or emotional problems. So while stress is often helpful, this chapter is concerned with *harmful* stress, the kind that can hurt you if it is not controlled.

WHAT CAUSES STRESS?

You may already be aware that any number of things can act as stressors. Work-related problems, marital disputes, family deaths, and many other situations—including many *positive* events—can cause stress. But in this book, we're most concerned with the effects of prostate cancer on your life, and prostate cancer can cause stress in a number of different ways. For example, pain can cause stress. Waiting for test results can cause stress. Concerns about how the cancer may affect you can cause stress. Worries about not being able to fulfill responsibilities can cause stress. Problems with treatments, adjustments to dietary changes, and fears of metastasis may also provoke a stress response.

Research has shown that the first one hundred days following a cancer diagnosis are particularly stressful. During this time, stress is most often caused by thoughts of life and death, although it may also involve fears about treatment and other aspects of the illness. Although stress does not go away completely after these first hundred days, it's comforting to know that it does diminish. (Remember, we're talking approximates here. Don't fall apart if you don't notice any change on day 101!)

So, certain events are likely to cause stress. But do these events by themselves cause stress? And will the events that cause stress in one person necessarily cause it in another person and cause it to the same degree? As you may have guessed, the answer is "No"! Why? Because every person has a unique way of responding to the world around him. Your pattern of response depends on a number of things. Your upbringing, your self-esteem, your beliefs about yourself and world, the way in which you guide yourself in your thoughts and actions—all of these things help determine your stress response. The degree to which you feel in control of your life also plays an important role in this response. And the way you feel physically and emotionally—as well as the way you get along with people—is also a factor.

To sum it up, everyone's method of dealing with stress is unique and individual, and depends on a complex combination of thoughts and behaviors. For simplicity, though, we can see the stress response as depending on the "chemistry" between two factors. The first factor is the stressor, or the outside pressure. In other words, what is going on around you that is creating a problem? The second factor is your interpretation of the event. It is the interaction of the stressor and your internal interpretation that determines your response to stress. (Sound familiar? Yes, it's the same "formula" that can be applied to anger, depression, and all other emotions.) So the "equation" for the stress response is as follows:

Stressor + Interpretation = Stress Response

This equation has important implications for coping with stress. Why? It shows you that stress is not solely the result of your environment, your illness, or any other factor around you. The way you interpret this stressor is of equal importance. Of course, some stressors would produce stress in anybody. What would happen, for example, if somebody pointed a knife at your throat? Calm acceptance, or a stress response? Get the point? In many situations, though, you do have the ability to control your reaction to the stressor.

As you learn about coping with stress, it's important to remember that your mind responds to any threats of stress as though they are real and happening right now. Any thoughts or images in your mind that produce a stress response are perceived as existing in the present, as the brain and the nervous system do not recognize the difference between past, present, and future. So it's easy to see that you contribute to your body's stress response with your thoughts and images. This makes it even more important to feed your mind with the best, the most beneficial, and the most constructive information available.

HOW CAN YOU COPE WITH STRESS?

Because stress can affect the body and mind in so many ways, stress management is a very important part of any program for coping with prostate cancer. We still don't know to what degree prolonged stress is involved in making the body more vulnerable to cancer. But we do know that stress can certainly play a role in exacerbating the unpleasant effects of prostate cancer. And we also know that the stress caused by cancer and its treatment is enormous on physical, social, and psychological levels. The good news is that regardless of how successfully you have dealt with stress in the past, you can learn effective strategies that will help you to deal with stress now. These strategies will make you feel more in control, lessening the feeling of panic, and increasing your emotional well-being. And because of the mind-body connection, these strategies will also help your body better cope with prostate cancer.

But before we look at how you should cope with stress, let's look at how you shouldn't cope with stress. Smoking, drinking alcohol, using inappropriate drugs, and overeating are all common but poor coping strategies. True, these activities will distract you and, perhaps, delay the effects of the stress, but they can also hurt you, and will prevent you from coping with stress in a constructive way.

So what should you do? Try to learn new, more appropriate ways of dealing with stress. Relaxation techniques and regular exercise can be helpful parts of stress-management programs. And by thinking more appropriately and more positively, you can go a long way toward reducing stress. But be realistic, and remember that stress can be managed and controlled, but it cannot be eliminated. Your focus, then, should be on using the following management techniques to help yourself deal better with both the physical and the emotional effects of the stress response.

Use Relaxation Techniques

Relaxation is incompatible with stress, so the best way to start controlling stress is to use relaxation techniques. In fact, relaxation techniques alone—used without any other coping strategies—may allow you to successfully cope with both the physical and emotional effects of stress.

Relaxation benefits you in many ways. First, it can give your body a chance to rest and recuperate. And a stronger body can help you deal better with the ravages of stress—and of life!—and may enable you to derive increased benefits from any medication you may be using. Relaxation will also help you sleep better. (Have you been experiencing any sleep problems since the onset of your prostate cancer?) Relaxation is also pleasurable, and will increase your feeling of emotional well-being. And relaxation can give you a powerful sense of reestablishing control over your life, despite the presence of a chronic medical problem. Relaxation helps you feel confident and competent.

There are many different types of clinical relaxation techniques, including meditation, autogenics, and deep breathing. Hypnosis and biofeedback can also be used to induce relaxation, although they have other uses, as well. (See Chapter 19 for a full discussion of these and other relaxation techniques.)

One relaxation technique that is often successful in combating stress is *imagery*—a technique that can also be used to cope with pain and other problems. Imagery is the process of formulating mental pictures or scenes in order to harness your body's energy and improve your physical or emotional well-being. In this case, of course, you'll want to conjure images that are relaxing and stress-free.

Alan was tense in anticipation of his radiation treatments, which would begin the next week. He was so tense, in fact, that he found it almost impossible to eat or sleep. Alan was instructed to get into a relaxed position in his favorite chair. The lights, he was told, should be dimmed, and all interruptions should be avoided. Alan imagined lying on a blanket at the beach. He felt the warmth of the sun and the caress of a gentle breeze on his legs. He heard the sounds of the waves lapping the shore, and the familiar call of sea gulls. He smelled the salt water and the suntan lotion. Soon, Alan began to relax. He relaxed so well, in fact, that he began to doze.

Of course, you'll want to imagine a scene that is particularly relaxing for you. Alan found the beach especially soothing. You may prefer another image. In order for this technique to work most effectively, try to make your images multisensory, as Alan did. In other words, imagine not only the sights, but also the smells, the tactile sensations (touch), and the sounds. The more vivid your image, the more helpful it will be. But feel comfortable with whatever degree of clarity your image takes on. The degree of relaxation you experience is up to you, and is of benefit to only you. You are in control.

Pinpoint the Source of Your Stress

Now that you're more relaxed, you're ready to objectively identify your stressors. What, specifically, is causing you to feel stress? Maybe you're having a hard time with the symptoms of prostate cancer. Maybe you're concerned about the reactions of others. Or maybe you're tired of thinking about cancer. These are all possible cancer-related stressors—and, of course, there are plenty more.

What if you're not sure what's causing your stress? Try keeping a log of your daily stressors. This will allow you to more easily see the people, places, and things that have the potential to create stress in your life. But what if you can't pinpoint which of your many activities are the real culprits? As you keep your log, you might want to use a numerical rating scale, such as the Subjective Units of Disturbance (SUD) Scale. How does it work? Ratings on this scale range from 0 to 100, depending on the amount of stress you're experiencing. Use 100 to represent the most extreme and disturbing stress, and 0 to represent no stress—total and complete relaxation. Then rate your activities, experiences, and thoughts. The ones with the higher SUD numbers are the ones causing you the most stress. For example, loud, blasting music from your neighbor's radio might be rated a whopping 85!

Identify Your Stress Reactions

Once you have begun identifying your stressors, you'll want to become completely aware of your responses to them. Are they more physiological or more psychological? What parts of your body seem to be the most vulnerable? What kinds of reactions does your body show? Does your attention span suffer? Do you get heart palpitations? Do you start losing confidence, or feel like you're "slipping"? As you become more aware of this, you will develop a complete picture of your unique stress response. This picture will help you choose the coping strategies that will be most useful in dealing with your stressors.

Eliminate Stressors When Possible

What's the next step? Once you recognize which stressors are causing the most trouble, try to determine whether or not you can eliminate them. Removing the source of the stress is an obvious and logical way to manage stress. For instance, if the task of managing your household expenses is causing you stress, you might have your wife or another member of your family take over this chore. Obviously, different types of stressors would have to be removed in other ways.

Change Your View of the Stressor

But what happens if you can't eliminate the source of your stress? You'll then have to work on your interpretation of the stressors. You might want to use some of the suggestions discussed in Chapters 11 and 13. Or you might want to try systematic desensitization, discussed in Chapter 12.

Another technique that might help you cope better with stressors is *stress inoculation*. How can you be inoculated against stress? Well, you're certainly familiar with the use of inoculations to protect children from disorders such as measles. By exposing a child to the virus or other agent that causes a disorder, inoculations gradually strengthen the child's immunity to the disorder. Similarly, stress inoculation uses mental rehearsal procedures to help you confront and gradually tolerate stressful situations. As we previously discussed, because your mind responds to thoughts and mental images as if they were real and happening right now, thinking about something can be just as stressful as experiencing it. So by learning to cope with a situation in your mind, you can learn how to cope with it before it even happens.

Start your stress inoculation process by using whatever relaxation techniques you have found most helpful. After you have achieved a comfortable level of relaxation, start imagining one of the stressors you've previously indicated. As you imagine the stressful scene, recognize any physiological sensations or psychological changes that you experience.

Jake realized that much of his stress was being caused by the fear that during an office visit, his doctor would tell him that his cancer had spread. Time and again, Jake's stress reaction—nausea and a tightening of the throat—would appear when he imagined this frightening scene. So Jake decided to use stress inoculation to gain control. Repeatedly, he imagined himself in the very situation he feared. He visualized the doctor's office. He imagined himself sitting in the chair by the doctor's desk. He actually heard the words he was afraid of. As Jake gradually increased his tolerance of this image of the dreaded event, the symptoms of his stress lessened.

Like Jake, every time you use stress inoculation to visualize and mentally experience a scene, you'll increase your ability to handle that particular stressor, and your symptoms will decrease. In other words, your body and mind will be "inoculated," allowing you to tolerate that stressor. An added advantage of using this technique is that you will become more aware of exactly when these tension-producing situations begin to affect you. This will enable you to use your coping strategies sooner, before your body and mind suffer from the stress response.

Don't feel that you have to use stress inoculation for every stressor you anticipate experiencing. And don't think you have to deal with every stressor all at once. Work with each scene until you feel that you've mastered it.

If you have already read the explanation of systematic desensitization found in Chapter 12, you may realize that stress inoculation and desensitization are very similar techniques. But there are differences. For instance, in desensitization, the technique of imagining a stressful situation is alternated with the use of relaxation techniques. In stress inoculation, relaxation techniques are employed only at the start of each session. In this case, it is simply repeated exposure to the stressor that puts you in control. Either—or both—of these techniques can help you cope with your emotions. Experimentation will show you which method is best for you.

Use Physical Stress Relievers

Certain physical activities can be great for stress control. For example, some people relieve tension or stress by driving. Certainly, as long as you continue to observe safety rules—and as long as you enjoy this activity—driving can be very relaxing. But if driving isn't your idea of a calming pastime, there are a number of other activities that may be just the ticket.

Exercise

Exercise is not only a wonderful means of releasing stress, but, as you'll learn in Chapter 22, it can be a very healthy component of any treatment program. Regardless of how prostate cancer is affecting you, there is certain to be a type of exercise that will help you control your level of stress. Brisk walking, swimming, and dancing, for instance, all allow for the release of tension. Just make sure to get your doctor's green light.

Keep Busy the Fun Way

Hobbies and other leisure activities are often very effective in reducing stress. Hobbies can divert your attention from the stressful situation, and direct it towards something more enjoyable. They may also help you feel productive—and a lack of productivity may be one of the stressors giving you problems in the first place! If you don't have a hobby, this is a great time to look into painting, model building, gardening—whatever suits your fancy. If you're already involved in a hobby, you now have the perfect reason to indulge yourself whenever you can.

Catch Up on Your Sleep

Another technique for dealing with stress is sleep. Some people have difficulty sleeping when they're experiencing high levels of stress. But, when possible, cat naps or even prolonged periods of sleep may help you reduce stress to a more manageable level.

A STRESSLESS SUMMARY

What are your goals? Are you trying to gain greater control over your emotions? Do you want to live life more fully? Whatever your goals may be, if stress is keeping you from reaching them, your stress response is negative. By learning how to control your stress—by eliminating the things that are stressing you, or by modifying your reaction—you'll be far more likely to meet these goals, and, just as important, you'll have a head start in coping successfully with prostate cancer.

Chapter 16

OTHER EMOTIONS

The emotions discussed in Chapters 9 through 15 are not the only ones you may experience, of course. Worry, for example, is a basic emotion. What might you worry about? Have you got a month to discuss all the possibilities? You might worry about the future, about how your life may change because of prostate cancer, and about countless other things.

What other emotions might you want to deal with better? This chapter will discuss four emotions that many men with prostate cancer have found problematic: boredom, envy, loneliness, and grief.

BOREDOM

Hopefully, by this time, you are not so bored that you have stopped reading! If I've still got your attention, let's talk a little about boredom.

What an empty feeling boredom is! It's one of the worst feelings you can experience. It has been said that more problems and tragedies are caused by boredom than by any other single condition.

Because you weren't born bored, you must have learned to be bored. And even now, you're not always bored. There are still certain things that hold your attention from time to time. Right? Let's talk about what might be causing your boredom, and see how you can better fight the boredom blues.

Is Prostate Cancer Boring You?

I bet you never thought of prostate cancer as being boring. But it can be because of the restrictions your condition may impose on you. Many activities that you enjoyed in the past may now seem to be out of reach. You may not even want to start something new, as you may feel that future activities will be too restricted by your condition.

So what should you do? Don't let your condition cause you to give up on life. Distinguish between what you can do and what you can't. If you do have to curtail some activities because of prostate cancer, you'll do so. If you have to drop an activity, you'll drop it. But don't eliminate all activities simply because you feel that you may not be able to complete them.

Try New Activities

Certainly, if boredom is a problem for you, you'll want to find ways to add some interest to your life. But don't feel that you must push yourself to enjoy something. Forcing yourself to be amused rarely works. You may find that the activities you used to enjoy now seem artificial and uninteresting. You may no longer get any pleasure from them. But this doesn't mean that you should give up on everything. What you want to do is to find some *new* activities that will make your life more interesting. Remember that preferences change. Be open-minded, and try things that never appealed to you before. This time, they may spark your interest.

Learn Something New

One of the most effective weapons against boredom is learning. The mind is like a thirsty sponge, always ready and willing to soak up more information and knowledge. Select a potentially interesting topic you don't know much about. Then go out and learn something about it. You may want to begin by simply going to the library and reading some books on the topic. Maybe you'd like to enroll in an adult education course. Often, boredom quickly disappears once you become involved in something new. As an added benefit, your new pursuit may put you in contact with some interesting new people. And increasing your circle of friends is a good way to fight boredom.

Set Goals

Boredom often arises from plodding along with no real purpose in life. So one of the best ways to fight boredom is to always give yourself something to look forward to—in other words, a goal. This doesn't mean that you'll never be bored again. You may still have to give yourself an occasional kick in the derriere to get yourself moving toward the goals you've chosen. But the promise of some pleasurable activity will make it much easier to keep yourself moving.

What kinds of goals might you set? Your goals can be as small and simple as reading a chapter of a good book, writing a letter, making that phone call you've been thinking about, watching a television program you enjoy, or meeting somebody special for lunch. Remember that your life is not over! Try to schedule something to look forward to every single day. This way, even if part of your day seems boring—because you're involved in household tasks, or because you have to rest to build up your strength—you won't give the weeds of boredom a chance to take root!

ENVY

You've heard the cliché, "The grass is always greener. . . ." If you have prostate cancer, you're probably envious of people who don't—people who feel well, and are able to do more than you can. This is understandable. But, while understandable, envy is a destructive emotion, because it's a type of self-torture. When you feel envious, you're constantly putting yourself down and comparing your own qualities with the seemingly better qualities of somebody else. You feel inferior. And this can lead to other negative emotions, such as anger or depression.

Often, envy is irrational. When you're envious, you want to be like somebody else. You want to have what somebody else has. Does this mean that the other person has a life that's happier than yours in every way? Stop and think for a moment. I'm sure you can come up with some areas in which your life is better!

What Leads to Envy?

Basically, there are four conditions necessary for envy to occur. First, you must feel deprived. You must feel as if you can't have something that you want or need. We're not talking simply about money, pleasure, or even health! Envy is an intense feeling that involves more than this. It seems as if your feeling of need lies deep inside.

Second, to experience envy, you must feel that somebody else has what you feel that you're missing. Perhaps that person has a bigger house, for instance. Or perhaps he has a "healthy" prostate.

Third, you must feel powerless to do anything about the problem. You must feel totally unable to change the circumstances that have made you envious in the first place. This helplessness causes you to feel more and more bitter. And this makes you even more envious!

Fourth, there must be a change in the relationship between you and the person whom you envy. You no longer simply compare yourself with the other person; you now feel fiercely competitive. You may begin to feel that the only reason you don't have what you want is that somebody else has it.

It's important to recognize that there are actually two types of things that may cause you to feel envy. One type is tangible—cars, boats, homes, friends, and so on. The other type is less tangible—pleasure or health, for instance. If you have prostate cancer, you may still have many tangible things. You may still have a car and a place to live. You may still have a job. But your medical condition may make you envious over less tangible things.

Make the Best of What You Have

To get rid of the destructive emotion called envy, concentrate on increasing those benefits and pleasures you *can* get out of life. Why worry about comparing yourself with somebody else? How is that going to help you? Sure, you may have cancer. But that doesn't mean you can't get a lot of enjoyment from life. Set up reasonable goals for yourself, considering what you *do* have and what you *can* do. Remember that you are who you are. Make the best of what your life has to offer.

LONELINESS

There is a difference between being alone and being lonely. Being alone simply means that there is no one else with you. This can be either good or bad. But being lonely is always negative. Loneliness is a sad, empty feeling in which you are upset by your awareness of being alone.

Why Are You Lonely?

Why might you feel lonely? You may feel left out if you can't spend time with others the way you used to—because you're not feeling well, perhaps. Or you may feel lonely because you think that other people don't understand your condition. You may simply feel different from others. And you may decide to change some of your relationships just because you're having a harder time dealing with people.

It's hard to be lonely—and not just because loneliness is such a bad feeling. You see, loneliness doesn't just happen. It actually takes effort to make yourself lonely and to keep yourself lonely. There are many opportunities to enjoy the company of others. As a result, loneliness usually occurs out of choice rather than accident. To be really lonely, you have to purposely exclude everyone around you from your life. You have to always be on your guard, protecting yourself from the horrible possibility of making new friends!

Do You *Want* to Be Lonely?

Why might you want to be lonely? There are four possible reasons. First, despite your complaints to the contrary, you may enjoy being lonely. In fact, you may enjoy it so much that you refuse to do anything about it. Why? Because you may feel more comfortable alone than you do in the company of others.

Second, if you're lonely, you may be hard to please. You may feel that you don't want to even bother trying to create new relationships because no one meets all of your requirements.

Third, you may feel that you must be lonely. You may have resigned yourself to it. You may tell yourself that this is an unavoidable part of having prostate cancer!

Fourth, and probably most important, if you're lonely, it may be because you're scared. You may be afraid of being rejected. You may recall previous relationships that did not work out the way you wanted, and feel that they are simply not worth the hurt and pain.

End Your Lonely Ways

Reading this isn't easy, especially if you are a lonely person. Why? It's not easy to think that you might have done this to yourself! But there is a light at the end of the tunnel! Recognize where your feelings of loneliness come from. Admit to yourself that it's not such a great feeling, and that you should try to change it. There are things you can do to fight loneliness.

Don't Be a Pusher

The first step in ending loneliness is to stop pushing people away. It's likely that you're giving off unseen vibrations—vibrations which tell people that you don't want them around. These vibrations can reduce your number of acquaintances, adding to your feeling of loneliness. This must stop. You have to learn to give off *positive* vibrations—the kind that welcome people instead of chasing them away. Smile at people. Show interest in what others have to say. Let people know that you like being with them.

Make Contact!

Once you start giving off new, more positive vibes, you'll want to make more friends. How can you meet people? You can start by getting involved in some kind of organization. Because you have prostate cancer, you may want to contact your local chapter of the American Cancer Society. There, you'll meet people with similar concerns. Besides relieving your loneliness, the members of your group may make you aware of valuable coping skills. You may even find ways of helping others.

If support groups are not your cup of tea, try getting involved in a new learning activity or hobby. Take adult education courses, for example. This may help alleviate loneliness as well as boredom. Invite people to your home. (Be sure to pace yourself so that you don't become exhausted.) Most important, be receptive to the people that you meet. Try to see the good in everyone. Don't reject someone simply because there are a few things about them that you don't like.

If you work at conquering loneliness, you'll feel much better about yourself and about your life. This will make life more enjoyable, even though you have prostate cancer. Give yourself and others a chance, and your feelings of loneliness will disappear, regardless of the limitations your condition has placed on you.

GRIEF

Grief is an unpleasant emotion. And feelings of grief—the mourning over a loss—are common to people who have prostate cancer, especially at the time of initial diagnosis.

Why Are You Grieving?

People grieve when they're aware that they've lost something that they value. In this case, you've lost your former lifestyle. This loss may be temporary or permanent. You may also feel that you have lost some physical strength. You may not like yourself as much, and may grieve over your damaged self-esteem. And if you are used to having one role within your family, and this role has been modified or significantly changed because of your medical condition, you may grieve this loss, as well.

Paul was a fifty-eight-year-old construction worker. He took pride in providing a good income for his wife and five children. Then prostate cancer came along. Now Paul was no longer able to work the overtime he had grown accustomed to. There was even a possibility that he would not be able to continue working in the construction field. And where else would he be able to earn that kind of money? Paul recognized that his wife would have to work to supplement his reduced income. Paul would no longer be the sole bread-winner, and he grieved this loss.

Certainly, Paul was miserable. But this does not mean that grief is bad. When the feeling of grief develops, it shows that something must be worked through before an adjustment can be made to the new situation—in this case, prostate cancer.

Combat Your Grief

What can you do about grief? Unfortunately, grief cannot be avoided. Only by analyzing your grief and working through it will you be able to get back to the act of living. Paul had to face the realities of his situation. He had to assess his abilities, and see what further skills might prepare him for less physically demanding work. Only by focusing on the source of his grief and beginning to address these concerns could Paul begin to feel better.

How else can you combat grief? Crying can be helpful, even if you don't think it's the "manly" thing to do. This doesn't mean that you should force yourself to sob, but if the tears start welling up, don't stop them. Let your feelings out. Think about what has changed and about what will change. Talk it out with the people you're close to. Don't avoid facing up to the fact that you have prostate cancer, as this denial will prevent you from going through the grief process.

Remember that grief is like a deep infection. The only way you can help certain infections get better is to open them up and let what's inside come out. This may be difficult, but eventually the wound will drain and begin to heal. Eventually, you will exhaust your grief. Then the healing will begin.

Living with any chronic medical problem can involve a number of painful emotions. But it is possible to cope with these emotions—to learn strategies that will eliminate or lessen them, and help you to live more comfortably and happily. These strategies are just what the doctor—and family and friends—ordered!

PART IV

CHANGES IN GENERAL LIFESTYLE

Chapter 17

COPING WITH LIFESTYLE CHANGES— AN INTRODUCTION

So you have to make changes in some aspects of your lifestyle because of prostate cancer? Yes, that is all part of the "package." But remember that throughout life, changes can occur for any number of reasons. If you began a new job, you might have to wake up at a different time, commute in a new direction using a different form of transportation, or adjust to a different salary. And if your new job required you to move, you would have to meet a whole new group of people.

In your case, it's prostate cancer that's a new part of your life. Although you may think that it will be impossible to lead a normal life knowing you have cancer, this isn't necessarily true. However, it is vital to give up the goal of avoiding change, and to concentrate on making changes that will allow you to lead a comfortable life despite prostate cancer. Remember that you want to feel better, to enjoy life, and to do what you can. These goals are both reasonable and achievable.

Prostate cancer can, to different degrees, affect work, family life, sexual activity, social activity, finances, and other aspects of day-to-day living. Make up your mind that any necessary changes will be worked through and accepted. But keep in mind that there are always things you can do to improve the way you live. Also keep in mind that your lifestyle will, to a large degree, be of your own choosing. You'll automatically take many different factors into consideration when determining what you want your lifestyle to be and how full you want your days to be.

You may decide to wait, to put things off—to avoid making any changes until you "feel better." But why wait? Why not try to see what you can do right now to improve the quality of your life, even while you're learning to live with prostate cancer?

MAKING CHANGES

A very important part of coping with prostate cancer is taking control over as much of your life as possible. This means taking an active part in making all treatment decisions, and determining how all aspects of treatment can fit as comfortably as possible into your lifestyle. Keep in mind that there's a difference between taking control of your life and looking for miracles. Yes, a miracle would be wonderful, but hoping for one will not help you improve your life. In fact, it might slow down your adjustment. So instead of looking for miracles, focus on doing the best you can to help yourself.

A diagnosis of prostate cancer may seem to be totally negative. However, this diagnosis can be positive if it serves as motivation for change or self-improvement. You see, people change and grow not only when things are going well, but also during times of adversity. By looking at your life from a different perspective, you may be able to start weeding out those things that have not been good for you and introducing better things. This will improve not only your own physical and emotional health, but also the well-being of those around you.

At this point, you want to change your lifestyle to make things as easy as possible for yourself. Appropriate changes can allow you to continue doing much of what you want to do without putting too much pressure on your body. In fact, as you modify your life to reduce or avoid discomfort and conserve energy, you should gradually feel better. For example, try spreading out your most taxing activities. Pace yourself. Make sure to include rest periods during the course of the day so you can "recharge your batteries." These changes should help you do many of the things you want to do while taking care of your physical needs. Below, you'll find other suggestions that may prove helpful.

Set Priorities

Look at yourself not as a person of limitless energy, but as one of limited energy. Focus on the most important things that you want to do in your life, and try to spend less time on things that don't have as much significance.

Each day, prioritize your activities so that you can spend your energy on those tasks and activities that are most important. Make up a list of the things that need doing, and then group them into "musts," "maybes," and "possibilities." On some days, you'll be able to do many of the things on the list; on other days, you may be able to do very few. During those times when you can do very few, you'll be glad that you were smart enough to accomplish the most important tasks first.

Just as you must accomplish certain tasks each day, you should also make it a point to do something you enjoy each day. Spend more time with those people and those activities that are more supportive of your physical and emotional well-being. Spend less time—or, possibly, no time!—with those people and activities that drain your strength and give you less pleasure. This will improve the overall quality of your life, better equipping you to deal with the stress of prostate cancer.

Despite all the changes you may be making because of your newly diagnosed condition, you want to maintain as much normalcy in your life as you can. Continue doing some of the things you're used to doing. Don't make too many changes, because if you do, you may lose track of what your life is all about.

As you work on modifying your lifestyle, also try to gradually modify your standards, requirements, and obligations. Don't feel that you have to live up to your previous standards—especially if your condition or treatment has diminished your strength. There is no law that says that you must keep your standards at the same level throughout your entire life. Be flexible and realistic, and change your criteria as needed to make yourself more comfortable.

Life with cancer can have its ups and downs. Changes may have to be made because of your emotional needs, your treatment, your symptoms, and other factors. The most efficient way to deal with these changes is to anticipate all the ups and downs and ride them out as smoothly as possible.

Set Goals

Always make sure you have something to live for. Life without goals is meaningless. Be sure to set short-term, intermediate-term, and long-term goals for yourself. For instance, you might choose the next book you'd like to read, find a new hobby or interest you'd like to pursue, or plan your next vacation. Then keep aiming towards these goals. This will put everything in your life in better perspective.

Live Life One Day at a Time

Live each day one day at a time. Although this may seem incompatible with having goals, it's not. You can continue to live one day at a time even though you have goals in the back of your mind to give your life focus. Enjoy life as much as you can. Try to add pleasure to some of the ordinary, mundane things that you previously gave little thought to. If you go for a ride in your car, for example, instead of focusing on your destination, enjoy the process of getting there. Look at the scenery around you. Admire the beautiful things that life has to offer.

GETTING USED TO CHANGES

What are some of the factors that will determine how well you'll adapt to the changes in your lifestyle? There are many. For example, what were you doing before you were diagnosed with prostate cancer? How satisfied were you with your work and leisure activities? How supportive were the people close to you—both family and friends? How has your condition affected you, both physically and emotionally? These and other factors will play a role in determining how you'll adjust to prostate cancer, its treatment, and any changes it necessitates. But that doesn't mean your hands are tied. You can improve the way you deal with virtually any factor.

At this point, your head may be spinning. You may fear that changes will have to take place in your activity schedule, your work life, and your social life. You may also be apprehensive about dealing with physical discomfort and medication. You may even worry that you won't be able to perform your normal chores and responsibilities. These concerns are in no way unusual. Most people with prostate cancer feel this way. But the fact that you can do much to improve your life should help you reduce your fears and approach change in a more positive way.

As you modify your lifestyle, be aware that the changes you make can affect your self-esteem. Your self-esteem is, to at least some degree, a reflection of the role you play in life: the way you deal with the people in your life, the activities you're involved in, and the routine that you follow. When any of these things changes, your self-esteem can change as well. By keeping this in mind, you may be more likely to make changes that will help you preserve—or improve!—your self-esteem.

What happens if you decide not to make necessary lifestyle changes? This may indicate that you're trying to deny your situation. As we discussed earlier in the book, denial is a very common coping strategy that can sometimes be positive. But it's important to be aware of its negative side, as well. What if denial keeps you from doing what you need to do? For example, what if you don't get enough rest, or you don't eat properly, or you don't follow your treatment regimen? This is destructive denial, and it can hurt you. Hopefully, the fact that you're reading this book in the first place shows that you're not really denying your condition. But continue to stay on top of this.

TREATMENT AND REHABILITATION

Coping with changes in lifestyle is a very important part of the process called *rehabilitation*. What is rehabilitation? Rehabilitation includes efforts designed to improve your physical condition, as well as your psychological, vocational, financial, and social well-being. And what is the goal of rehabilitation? To enable you to function at the best level possible, allowing for any changes that must be made because of the effects of cancer and its treatment. Another name for rehabilitation might be readaptation, since the goal is to help you become incorporated once again in the mainstream of society.

What Are the Four Types of Rehabilitation?

There are four general categories of cancer rehabilitation.

Preventative rehabilitation, the first type, is used when you anticipate experiencing certain disabilities because of your cancer and its treatment. As part of preventative rehabilitation, education or special training may help you to minimize the impact of these disabilities. (For information on special training, see Chapter 23.)

Restorative rehabilitation helps you to physically return to the way you were before you had prostate cancer—or, at least, to come as close as possible to that state. For example, if a radical prostatectomy leaves you unable to have an erection, a penile implant could enable you to once again have sex. (For information about sex and prostate cancer, see Chapter 31.)

Supportive rehabilitation uses a support network to help you deal with any permanent or disabling problems resulting from your treatment. The goal, of course, is to enable you to function as normally as possible. (For information on support groups, see Chapter 9.)

Palliative rehabilitation is used when the cancer is so advanced that it is unlikely that there will be a recovery. Palliative efforts—the use of painkillers, for example—are therefore designed to provide as much comfort and emotional support as possible, so that you can still participate in as much day-to-day activity as your condition permits. (For information on medication, see Chapter 18.)

Who's Involved in Rehabilitation?

In general, cancer rehabilitation uses a team approach so that different people are available to help you with different facets of your life. Who does this team include? Well, the most important person, of course, is you! Add to that your family and friends, as well as professionals dealing with both the body and the mind. And which professionals may be involved in such a team? In addition to your oncologist or urologist and your primary physician, you may want to include specialists from the fields of nursing, nutrition, psychology, physical therapy, occupational therapy, and, perhaps, religion. You may also want to include an attorney and a financial adviser.

In many cases, the hospital that you are working with will have a network of all the medical professionals you'll need on your team. However, not all hospitals have such teams set up. In this case, you may want your physician to help you coordinate the formation of your rehabilitation team.

GUIDELINES FOR CHANGE

There are a number of things that you can do to make any changes necessitated by your condition easier and more comfortable. The following are some general guidelines for living with prostate cancer.

☐ Make your house user-friendly. Where you have potentially dangerous conditions—steps, tile floors, and so on—be sure to install guardrails, grab bars, and no-slip floor coverings. Every bit of energy that you conserve by making things easier for yourself around the house—and this includes appliances, structural changes, clothing modifications, and more—can be funneled into areas that will better enhance your overall lifestyle.

☐ If your mobility is limited—or if you anticipate that it will be limited, even temporarily—obtain a handicapped parking permit from your local department of motor vehicles. In most cases, you'll have to get a letter from your doctor saying that this is necessary. It may take time to get this permit, so act now so that the permit will be ready when you need it.

☐ Make sitting more comfortable by using the special foam mattresses sometimes referred to as "egg crate" mattresses. Use them as pads on your bed or cut them into pillows. They're light enough to be moved around the house as needed.

☐ Build up a supply of loose-fitting jogging suits, sweat suits, and other types of comfortable clothing—clothing that is nonbinding and easy to put on and take off. Velcro fasteners will make it easier to open and close your garments.

☐ Consider getting a cordless phone if you're going to be alone for any period of time. This will enable you to always have a phone on hand.

☐ Be aware of how your body feels—how it reacts to different activities. Then act accordingly, resting as necessary.

☐ Build on the talents and activities you can still enjoy—and there are sure to be plenty of them! Try to focus on the things that you still have, rather than the things that you have lost. This guideline can be applied to relationships, activities, abilities, and interests.

☐ Give yourself permission to indulge in the things you enjoy. There are probably enough negative things in your life right now! Allow yourself to enjoy the positive things without guilt.

☐ Pamper yourself a little, and learn that you don't have to do everything yourself. Accept help from others when necessary, and don't overextend yourself.

☐ Simplify your life. Work to reduce the pressures that you place on yourself by focusing on the tasks that must be done and temporarily shelving those tasks that are less urgent.

☐ Be more protective of yourself. Establish and follow routines that will supply you with the proper amounts of sleep, exercise, and nutrition. Take the precautions necessary to guard against accidents and infections.

☐ Improve your ability to communicate. Problems in communication are the main cause of the breakdown of relationships. By improving your communication, not only will you decrease the chances that your existing relationships will fall apart, but you'll also increase the likelihood of establishing new, more enjoyable relationships.

☐ Maintain control over your life, and do as much as you can—without exhausting yourself, of course. Research has suggested that people who maintain as many of their normal routines and activities as possible feel better and recover faster.

What's the best approach to making lifestyle changes? Always remember that you are the most important ingredient in the recipe for successful adjustment. So do everything you can to help yourself. All of your efforts are sure to reap invaluable benefits in the form of greater health and happier day-to-day living.

AS WE MOVE ON

Yes, you may have to make some changes in your lifestyle. But why assume that all of them will be negative? Isn't it possible that some of them will be for the better? Maybe you've been such a hard worker that you've never spent enough time with your family. If you have to cut back on your work schedule because of prostate cancer, perhaps you'll truly enjoy the increased time you'll be able to to spend with your wife or children. It's even possible that some of the medications you'll use to control prostate cancer will help control other pesty problems that have been troubling you for a while, whether or not the problems are related to prostate cancer. Certainly, learning to take better care of yourself will pay off in the long run. So, as you modify your lifestyle, be sure to look for the positive.

In the remaining chapters of Part IV, we'll look at positive modifications that will allow you to better cope with pain, fatigue, and other effects of prostate cancer and its treatment. We'll also look at diet, exercise, medication—in other words, at many of your lifestyle concerns. So read on, and let's get your act together!

Chapter 18

MEDICATION

Lifestyle changes, an improved mental attitude, dietary modifications, sufficient rest, and appropriate exercise—topics that will be discussed later in Part IV—are all good means of dealing with any physical and emotional problems related to prostate cancer. But these techniques may not always be enough. In this case, it may be beneficial to use another common adjunct to prostate cancer treatment—medication.

Certainly, attitudes vary concerning the use of medication. Some people welcome drugs as a powerful means of controlling physical or emotional problems. Others are afraid of their power, and of eventually becoming dependent on them. Still others resent the presence of any artificial substance in their body. Where do your feelings fit in?

Because of the possible side effects of many medications, it is certainly more desirable to treat prostate cancer without drugs. But there may be cases in which you and your physician feel that your symptoms warrant the use of medication. If so, it is essential to take the prescribed medications according to your doctor's orders. Do not play with medications that haven't been prescribed—or, for that matter, with ones that *have* been prescribed.

So let's talk more about medications so that if you do need them, you'll be able to cope with them, maximizing safety and effectiveness, and minimizing side effects.

CHOOSING THE APPROPRIATE MEDICATION

How does a doctor determine which medication should be used? In prescribing a drug program, your physician will take into consideration the severity of your condition, as well as the symptoms you're experiencing, any other drugs you may be taking, your age, and your overall health, among other factors. Certainly, if, in the past, you have shown sensitivities to any drugs, you should let your doctor know this—even if you think that this information is already part of your medical record.

The more facts your doctor has on hand, the better chance he or she will have of finding the right treatment for you.

Although many factors are considered before a medication is prescribed, your doctor cannot be sure exactly how a given medication will affect you. So, in many cases, trial-and-error will be necessary to determine the best drug and dosage for you. This can be frustrating, but keep in mind that the right drug—or combination of drugs—may greatly increase your level of comfort. So try to be patient!

KNOWING HOW AND WHEN TO TAKE YOUR MEDICATION

Whenever your doctor prescribes a medication, be sure you understand exactly what the medication is supposed to do, and how and when it should be taken. For example, certain medications should be taken only after meals, while others must be taken on an empty stomach. In still other cases, specific foods must be avoided during drug therapy.

Each person has different needs as far as dosage and frequency are concerned. Even if somebody you know has the same symptoms that are troubling you and is taking the same medication, his dosage may not necessarily be appropriate for you. And once you start taking the medication, your dosage may be adjusted based on any side effects you're experiencing and how well the medication is managing your symptoms.

Very few physicians will keep you on high doses of any medication unless they feel it's absolutely essential. Still, if you're taking a substantial amount of any drug and you question the need for such a dose, don't be afraid to ask your doctor about it. Every good doctor should be willing and able to explain your program. If you're feeling good, and you would like to reduce your dosage—or stop taking the drug altogether—by all means, speak to your doctor. Together, you will be able to plan a schedule for reducing your dosage and, if possible, ending treatment.

THEY MIGHT NOT GET ALONG

Never take any medications other than those prescribed for you without first checking with your doctor. If you need to take many different pills, it's important to avoid playing with your dosage, playing with the times you take the medications, or moving around the number of pills you take at a particular time. Follow your doctor's prescription as carefully as possible.

If you go to physicians other than the one who's handling your prostate cancer, be aware that they may prescribe medications that absolutely should not be taken with your prostate cancer medications.

The advantage of having one primary physician in charge of your care is obvious. Any other doctor you need can then consult with your primary physician to make sure that the treatment strategies will work together, rather than worsening your condition. Because certain medications are chemically incompatible, you should never mix drugs without knowing that the combination is safe. Don't take the chance. Check it out. And always make sure that each of the doctors you're working with knows all of the medications you're taking.

SIDE EFFECTS

Very likely, you are concerned about the possible side effects of any prescribed medication. Side effects, as you know, are the less-than-pleasant effects a drug may have on your body. Nausea, dry mouth, discolored urine, increased or reduced appetite, sleep disorders—these are all possible side effects. In fact, side effects are probably one of the biggest concerns about medication.

Because medication causes chemical changes within the body, side effects may occur whenever a drug is taken. And, unfortunately, the more powerful the drug, the more potent the side effects may be. If the side effects you experience are slight, you will probably want to ignore them—especially if the medication you're taking is having the desired effect. Even if the side effects are disturbing, you may want to take the medication if its benefits outweigh any discomforts you're experiencing. However, if side effects are having a particularly harsh impact on you, your physician should be informed, and the two of you should weigh the disadvantages against the advantages. In fact, *any* side effects should be reported to your doctor so that he or she can determine if the drug therapy should be continued, changed, or ended.

With any drug, it's important to find the lowest effective dose. This is one way to maximize the productivity of the medication and, hopefully, minimize any side effects. Side effects may also be minimized by taking the medication exactly the way it's been prescribed for you. (Again, if there are problems, call your doctor!)

GETTING DOWN TO SPECIFICS

In Chapter 7, we discussed the medications used in hormone therapy. But there are three other categories of medication that may be used in the treatment of prostate cancer: antianxiety drugs, antidepressants, and pain medications. As you read the following discussion, you'll see that there are several drugs in each category. Although they may generally work in the same way, there are at least minor differences between these drugs. Why is this important? If the prescribed medication has an unpleasant side effect, another drug from the same category may be able to give you the same benefits *without* the side effects. And if the prescribed drug is not making you feel better, another medication may do the trick. Your doctor will work with you to find the medication that works best with your particular chemistry.

So let's look at the drugs most commonly used to control anxiety, relieve depression, and reduce pain.

Antianxiety Medications

Much attention has been given to the anxiety and panic that often accompany medical problems such as prostate cancer. Many people have been able to reduce these symptoms through nonpharmacological methods—relaxation techniques, exercise, and other stress-management strategies. (See Chapter 12 for more about anxiety.) But if medication seems to be the answer for you—and especially if you've been experiencing panic attacks—there are three subcategories of drugs that may be helpful.

The first subcategory of the antianxiety drugs is the benzodiazepines. The drugs in this group include Xanax (alprazolam), as well as several others that have been effective in helping people deal with panic. These medications are similar to Valium (diazepam) and Librium (chlordiazepoxide hydrochloride), which, although also able to control anxiety, are not considered panic-attack medications. The benzodiazepines have few side effects, but can be habit-forming.

The second subcategory of drugs primarily used in the treatment of panic is the tricyclic antidepressants. These medications were actually among the earliest ones found effective in dealing with panic, but are now used less often, since more effective medications have been found. The drugs in this category include Tofranil (imipramine hydrochloride) and Norpramin (desipramine hydrochloride).

The third subcategory of antianxiety drugs is the MAO (monoamine oxidase) inhibitors. Some consider this group to be the most effective for panic control. However, of the three groups, this one probably requires the greatest care in following dosage schedules and other precautions in order to minimize side effects. For example, if you're taking a MAO inhibitor, it is important to avoid taking antihistamines or decongestants, as the drugs might be incompatible and cause further problems. Also, foods with high concentrations of tyramine or dopamine—aged cheeses, beer, and wine, for instance—should be avoided, as they may lead to hypertension (high blood pressure). Examples of drugs in this subcategory are Nardil (phenelzine sulfate) and Parnate (tranyl-cypromine sulfate).

When using antianxiety medications, keep in mind that even when they are effective, they are really only blocking the panic attacks. It is still important to deal with the triggers of the panic attacks, and to implement any changes necessary to resolve the problems that led to the anxiety in the first place.

Antidepressants

Unfortunately, depression is a common problem for people with prostate cancer. As discussed in Chapter 11, nonmedical coping techniques often can successfully deal with depression. When problems persist, though, a number of different antidepressants, including the tricyclics and MAO inhibitors mentioned in the previous section, may prove helpful. These medications work in different ways, and result in different possible side effects. Examples of other antidepressants include Desyrel (trazodone hydrochloride), Elavil (amitriptyline hydrochloride), Ludiomil (maprotiline hydrochloride), Pamelor (nortriptyline hydrochloride), Prozac (fluoxetine hydrochloride), and Sinequan (doxepin hydrochloride).

Pain Medications

As you'll discover when you read Chapter 19, several different types of techniques can be used to control pain. Medications are especially helpful in the treatment of nonlocalized (general) pain.

There are a number of categories of pain-control medications, also called analgesics. Two of the simplest nonnarcotic pain relievers are aspirin (acetylsalicylic acid) and Tylenol (acetaminophen). These medications can be very effective in relieving mild to moderate pain. Aspirin can also reduce swelling and inflammation, but may affect the stomach and can interfere with blood clotting. Therefore, Tylenol, while it doesn't control inflammation, may be preferred by some individuals.

Nonsteroidal anti-inflammatory drugs, another type of nonnarcotic analgesic, include over-the-counter drugs such as nonprescription-strength Motrin (ibuprofen), Advil (ibuprofen), and Nuprin (ibuprofen); and prescription medications such as prescription-strength Motrin (ibuprofen), Naprosyn (naproxen), and Indocin (indomethacin).

Narcotic pain relievers are much more powerful than the nonnarcotic analgesics. Narcotics, which are derived from opium or synthetically produced to act like drugs derived from opium, work by changing one's perception of pain and causing a heightened sense of well-being. Unfortunately, these drugs can also be habit-forming, and frequently cause side effects, including nausea, vomiting, or drowsiness. Examples of narcotic painkillers include codeine, Demerol (meperidine hydrochloride), morphine sulfate, Percodan (oxycodone/aspirin), Percocet (oxycodone/acetaminophen), and Darvon (propoxyphene hydrochloride). These medications may be used by themselves or in combination with over-the-counter pain relievers.

Analgesics can be administered orally, in pill or liquid form; by injection; through rectal suppository; or in an intravenous drip. Pain medication can also be delivered using a pain pump, also called a medication pump, which can be either implanted or worn next to the body. The pain pump is commonly used to allow the self-administration of prescribed doses of powerful, fast-acting painkillers.

Any time you deal with painkillers—as well as many other types of drugs—you have to be concerned about addiction. In fact, some people who have pain are reluctant to use painkillers because they fear addiction, or because they worry that other people will think less of them for using these drugs. In general, specialists report that addiction is rarely a problem in individuals with cancer. Why? Because pain medication is usually used only when necessary, with the least-powerful drugs being used whenever possible. When the medication is no longer needed, use of the drug is discontinued.

CAUTION!

There is always the chance that certain drugs—including over-the-counter drugs—may not be appropriate in your fight against prostate cancer. You've heard this a lot already, but it's important: Check with your doctor! Question, learn, and help yourself. Consult with your physician before taking even the most innocent-seeming over-the-counter drug. You never know when you might have a bad reaction.

In addition, be careful about bad mixes. This is so important that it bears repeating. For example, tranquilizers and alcohol should never be taken at the same time. Many mixes can make your symptoms worse, interfere with the action of the prescribed medication, or cause additional problems. Again, don't hesitate to ask questions!

WORK WITH YOUR PHARMACIST

Many people rely solely on their doctor for information about prescribed medications. If this is true of you, you're overlooking a great information resource: your pharmacist. Frequently, pharmacists know even more than physicians do about drug interactions, about which foods should be avoided when taking certain medications, and about other possible problems. So it can be helpful to develop a good working relationship with your local pharmacist, and to go to that same pharmacist for all your medications.

Besides being a source of information about drug actions, your pharmacist may be able to help you reduce costs. How? He or she may be able to suggest a less-expensive brand-name or generic drug. While there may be nothing wrong with the substitute drug, in some cases, certain formulations may work better than others. So always make sure to consult your physician before changing brands. (Depending on how your doctor filled out the prescription, your pharmacist may *have* to contact your doctor before substituting any brand other than the one specified.) Obviously, a good relationship with a well-informed, helpful pharmacist may benefit you in more ways than one.

ADDITIONAL MEDICATION 'MINDERS

Once you've begun taking a medication, make sure to let your physician know if the drug is having the desired effect. Any significant changes in your health, whether good or bad, should be reported to your physician. In this way, your doctor will be able to make an informed decision about whether your current drug plan should be continued or changed.

If you find that you're having trouble remembering to take your medication—or if you're sometimes not sure if you've already taken a dose—find ways to keep track of your medication schedule. For instance, you might prepare a daily chart that lists each dose separately. This will allow you to check off each dose as you take it. You might also purchase one of the new multi-compartment pill boxes, some of which can store a week's worth of drugs, divided into appropriate days and times. Some sophisticated devices even sound an alarm when the time comes for you to pop your pill!

Keep a list in your wallet of the medications you take. Show the list to your doctor, your pharmacist, or anyone else who needs to know what you're taking. (Makes for great "show and tell" at the corporate board meetings!)

You may experience certain emotional reactions to taking medication, such as depression or anger. These emotions should be coped with as soon as possible, before they adversely influence your physical and emotional well-being. If necessary, look back at the chapters on coping with emotions. If the suggested coping strategies don't provide relief, by all means seek out a qualified professional who can help you become more comfortable with your treatment plan.

A FINAL PRESCRIPTION

Many types of drugs other than those mentioned in this chapter may also be helpful for individuals with prostate cancer. In fact, there are so many possible combinations of drugs that it may take your doctor time to determine the "formula" that's best for you.

Hopefully, the information presented in this chapter has given you a good idea of what you must know in order to use medication as safely and effectively as possible. So if your doctor prescribes something new, ask about it. Not only will you probably feel a lot better as a result of taking the medication, but you'll know *why* you're feeling better!

Chapter 19

PAIN

Ouch! (Just getting you ready for this chapter!) Might you experience pain with prostate cancer? Unfortunately, sometimes. Pain is common when prostate cancer spreads to the bones or affects urination. In some cases, in fact, bone pain is what first brings individuals to the doctor for diagnosis.

When most people think about cancer, they think about pain. Pain—especially uncontrollable and intolerable pain—is probably one of the most frightening aspects of cancer. However, while some people with prostate cancer experience some type of pain, you might not experience the degree of pain that you fear, and it's very possible that any pain you do experience can be very well controlled. In many cases, once the specific type, location, and degree of pain has been diagnosed, regular intervention, in the form of medications or other techniques, may even prevent the recurrence of pain.

Pain prevention can be a very important part of cancer treatment. Chronic pain can weaken the body, leaving you vulnerable to further problems. By controlling or eliminating pain, you will strengthen your body and enhance your well-being.

When coping with pain, it's first necessary to identify the cause of the pain. Once this is done, treatment can often be aimed at eliminating the cause. But there's a problem. In some cases, it may be impossible to do anything about the underlying cause. In these instances, the pain itself, rather than the cause of the pain, is the most important concern.

Let's learn more about pain—why it occurs, and what treatments can be effective in its control.

WHEN AND WHY DOES PAIN OCCUR?

Pain is a message sent from your body to your brain saying that something is wrong. This painful signal begins when tissue is damaged or hurt. An electrical impulse is sent through the spinal cord to the sensory center of the brain, called the *thalamus*. Then the signal goes to the brain's outer layer, the *cortex*. When the message is received in the cortex, you're able to determine the location of the pain and its intensity. Signals are then sent from the brain back through the spinal cord, triggering the release of natural painkillers such as *endorphins*—the body's own "morphine." This often diminishes the pain.

There are a number of reasons why pain may occur in individuals with prostate cancer. For instance:

- [ ] Inflammation or tumor growth may irritate or place pressure on nerve endings.
- [ ] The tumor may obstruct hollow areas—areas with no organs or other structures—eventually pressing on adjacent structures.
- [ ] Cancer cells may metastasize to the bones.
- [ ] Bones may fracture as a result of metastasis.
- [ ] Cancer cells may block blood vessels, reducing blood circulation.
- [ ] Inactivity caused by prostate cancer may lead to stiffness.
- [ ] Treatments such as radiation or hormone therapy may cause painful constipation, nerve damage, inflammation, or muscular problems.
- [ ] Tumor-released chemicals may act on the nervous system.

Although pain may initially be physical, emotions can quickly worsen any pain you perceive. Anxiety or boredom, for example, can cause pain to appear more pronounced. Stress can cause muscles to tense, also increasing the degree of pain. Depression, too, may cause you to feel more pain, as it increases the tendency to focus on pain. And, of course, any pain you feel may increase the degree to which you experience anxiety, stress, or depression, which can lead to more pain, creating a vicious cycle.

Other factors, too, may exacerbate the pain. For instance, fatigue may worsen pain by preventing your tissues from getting the rest they need to repair themselves. Your perception of pain may also vary based on your own tolerance, as well as the degree to which you think the pain can be controlled. So, you see, the experience of pain is highly subjective, and is affected by many factors. You'll want to try to control some or all of these factors in order to manage your pain more successfully.

TREATMENT FOR PAIN

How can you start to deal with pain? Keep track of when the pain occurs, how often it occurs, how long it lasts, and how intense it is. This will help you decide if the pain is something you can handle yourself, or if it's serious enough to be brought to your doctor's attention. Remember: If in doubt, check it out. Inform your doctor about the pain. Together you can work out the best way of dealing with it.

If you decide that medical treatment is necessary, try to provide your doctor with an accurate description of the pain. Explain the location of the pain, how long you've had it, and whether the sensation is steady, sharp, throbbing, or dull. Also describe the intensity of the pain, whether mild, moderate, or severe, and discuss anything that seems to relieve the pain, as well as other symptoms that accompany the pain. The doctor should also be made aware of any treatments you have already tried for pain relief, whether or not these treatments were successful. Remember that health-care professionals have no way of knowing how severe your pain is unless you tell them, so don't be afraid to let them know how you feel.

Why is it so important for the doctor to understand the nature of the pain you're experiencing? Only by knowing all the facts will the doctor be able to determine the type of medication or other technique that is most appropriate in your case. You see, you'll want to use a medication or procedure that will be compatible with the type of pain you're experiencing.

Three general categories of treatment are used in the control of prostate-cancer pain: medical treatment (medication, radiation, or nerve blocks); physical therapy; and psychological strategies. All three types of therapies work by interrupting the transmission of pain messages before the brain receives and interprets them. Let's see how these three approaches can help you control—or, ideally, eliminate—pain.

Medical Treatment

In the medical treatment of prostate cancer, three different techniques may be used to control pain: radiation, medication, and nerve blocks. Your doctor's choice of treatment will depend partly on the nature and location of the pain, and, of course, partly on your previous responses to pain-control techniques.

When pain is localized—when it's experienced in the bones, for instance—low-level radiation treatments often work quickly and effectively, providing long-lasting relief. Two areas in which radiation has proven especially helpful are the hips and the pelvic region. (See Chapter 6 for more information on radiation.)

When pain is not localized, medication may be used to provide relief. In the case of mild pain, aspirin and other anti-inflammatory drugs may prove helpful. When pain is more severe, however, stronger drugs may be used to decrease or eliminate the pain. (For more information on medications, see Chapter 18.)

When using medication to control the pain of prostate cancer—or to control any pain—it's wise to remember that these drugs work by blocking pain signals. This can be dangerous when the medication blocks messages that would otherwise tell you about further metastasis or other problems.

When the pain of prostate cancer is extreme, a nerve block may be used to provide either temporary or permanent relief. This procedure involves injecting an anesthetic such as cortisone or alcohol into or around the nerve. In some drastic cases, nerves may be cut or destroyed to permanently eliminate feeling—and, therefore, pain—in the affected area.

Sometimes, radiation, medication, and nerve blocks fail to eliminate all the pain. In these cases, physical or psychological treatments may help. Let's learn more about these therapies.

Physical Therapy

The localized pain of prostate cancer can often be effectively relieved with one or more types of physical therapy, including TENS units, heat, cold, massage, and acupuncture. By pinpointing the location, frequency, and intensity of the pain, professionals can determine which type of physical therapy is most likely to be of help.

TENS (transcutaneous electric nerve stimulation) units can be helpful in dealing with localized pain. With this technique, electrodes are placed on the skin and joined to a machine with wires. Electric signals are then sent to the nerve endings, blocking the pain signals before they reach the brain. This method is safe, has no known side effects, and is not considered painful, although some people have reported mild feelings of discomfort. Pain relief from TENS therapy can be long- or short-term in nature.

Heat is another effective means of reducing pain, especially muscle soreness. Try applying heat with a hot water bottle, an electric heating pad, or a wet towel. Hot baths or showers may also be helpful. Just be sure to take any precautions necessary to avoid burns. For instance, do not use a heating pad on high for a long period of time, and do not allow yourself to fall asleep while using the pad.

Cold is often more effective than heat, providing faster and longer-lasting relief. Gel packs, which can be obtained from pharmacies and medical supply stores, are an effective means of applying cold, and, because of their pliable consistency, are often more comfortable than ice packs. These gel packs are kept in the freezer, removed for use, and then refrozen. Of course, if you don't have a gel pack, ice cubes placed in a plastic bag can be just as effective. Be sure to wrap either of these applications in a towel before holding them on the skin. Professionals usually advise you to apply an ice or other cold pack for twenty minutes, to remove it for twenty minutes, and to keep alternating periods of use and rest for as long as desired.

Massage can be used on the painful area itself or on the surrounding area. This technique can be performed by a professional, or you can perform it yourself, provided that the area is accessible to you and that you can use the technique effectively. By all means, check with a physician or physical therapist before attempting to employ massage as a means of controlling your pain.

Another type of physical therapy—one that has gained increasing use by professionals in the last few years—is *acupuncture*. This ancient Chinese technique involves the insertion of very thin needles into the body at specific points predetermined to bring about pain relief. These needles are inserted at various depths and angles, and are said to affect nerves in a way that suppresses pain perception. The needles may also trigger the release of endorphins, the body's natural painkillers. In fact, in China, acupuncture is often used as an anesthetic during surgery, indicating a high degree of effectiveness in many cases.

Although the insertion of needles may sound painful, patients rarely experience anything more than occasional, temporary discomfort when undergoing acupuncture therapy. If you are interested in trying acupuncture, speak to your physician or physical therapist, who should be able to guide you to a qualified professional.

As you can see, several physical therapy techniques can be used at home, whenever pain relief is needed. And all techniques are safe and without side effects when used correctly. You can further enhance the effectiveness of these techniques by making sure that you get the proper balance of rest and exercise.

Psychological Techniques

As we discussed earlier in the chapter, there are many factors that may influence your experience of pain, including anxiety, depression, and stress. When you learn to control these factors, you're sure to feel a lot better. This is not to say that the pain is "all in your head." But pain is usually a combination of physiological and psychological factors. So although you may be experiencing true physiological pain, your mind is very much involved in determining exactly how much it hurts.

What does all this mean? If medication, radiation, nerve blocks, and various physical therapies don't alleviate your pain, you can still relieve some—if not all—of it by working on your mind's *perception* of the pain. Many people have found effective pain control through the use of relaxation techniques, imagery, hypnosis, and biofeedback. These techniques work by separating you from your sensations of pain, enabling you to feel better. Some of these techniques may be learned at home. Others must be taught by professionals. The following discussions should help you decide which of the psychological pain-control techniques may best help you as you learn to cope with prostate cancer.

Relaxation Techniques

As discussed earlier, tension can actually increase your pain. So it makes sense that relaxation—the opposite of tension—can help you reduce your overall level of pain. As an added benefit, relaxation techniques may increase your general sense of well-being and help you deal better with many day-to-day problems—not just those problems related to prostate cancer.

In Chapter 15, you learned how imagery may be used to induce relaxation. Other types of relaxation procedures include progressive relaxation, meditation, autogenic training, deep breathing, and a method that I call the Quick Release. Let's look briefly at each of these techniques.

Progressive relaxation is based on the premise that when you experience anything stressful, the body responds with muscle tension—which, of course, can increase pain. In this procedure, which is usually performed for fifteen to twenty minutes once or twice daily, you sequentially tense and then relax the different muscle groups in your body, one group at a time. Most likely, you're already familiar with this popular and effective technique. If you wish to learn more, don't hesitate to consult books at your local library or speak to a professional.

Meditation can allow you to achieve a deep level of relaxation in a short period of time. During meditation, you focus your mind, uncritically, on one object, sound, activitiy, or experience, and "clear out" any extraneous thoughts. This technique, depending on the type of meditation you choose to use, works best when taught by a professional or learned from a reliable book.

Autogenics is a systematic program that helps you to train your body and mind to respond to your own verbal commands to relax. With this procedure, which can be used for short periods of time and repeated as frequently as needed, you give yourself verbal suggestions of heaviness, warmth, and calmness. Again, a book on relaxation techniques or a qualified professional can guide you in the use of this procedure.

Many people find that *deep breathing* can significantly increase their relaxation, and, as a result, decrease their pain. Deep breathing can be used in a number of different ways. Let's try one simple deep-breathing exercise together. First, assume a comfortable position on your bed or on the floor. Then put one hand on your abdomen and the other on your chest. Then inhale slowly and deeply through your nose, so that the hand on your abdomen moves higher. Hold your breath as long as you're comfortable doing so; then exhale slowly through your mouth, making a peaceful whooshing sound. Feel the hand on your abdomen sink slowly, and allow a growing feeling of relaxation to deepen inside you. Repeat this sequence for five to ten minutes. Then give yourself a few minutes to become aware of your surroundings before you get up. Practice this technique at least twice a day, extending its length if you wish.

Another simple but effective relaxation technique I call the *Quick Release*. Read the directions first, and then try it. Close your eyes, take a deep breath, and hold your breath as you tighten the muscles in every part of your body that you can think of—your fists, arms, legs, stomach, neck, buttocks, etc. Continue to hold your breath and keep your muscles tense for about six seconds. Then let your breath out in a "whoosh," and allow the tension to drain out of your muscles. Let your body go limp. Keep your eyes closed, and breathe rhythmically and comfortably for about twenty seconds. Repeat this tension-relaxation cycle three times. By the end of the third repetition, you'll probably feel a lot more relaxed. Keep practicing this technique, as constant practice will condition your body to respond quickly and completely.

Many other relaxation techniques may also prove helpful. Remember that your ability to increase relaxation and decrease pain by means of the mind-body connection are limited only by your imagination. Don't overlook this valuable way of improving your well-being.

Imagery

Much research has indicated that bodily functions previously thought to be totally beyond conscious control can be modified using psychological techniques. Imagery, a technique that has grown in popularity in the last several years, uses this mind-body connection to help you cope with disease.

Imagery is the process of conjuring up mental pictures or scenes in order to better harness your body's energy. In practice, imagery has been beneficial in helping people deal with a host of physiological and psychological problems. In addition to reducing stress, imagery has been successful in the control of headaches, hypertension, depression, and pain. Sometimes used alone, imagery can also be used in combination with prescribed medical treatment.

How can you use imagery to control the pain of prostate cancer? Get into a relaxed position in a comfortable chair or in bed. The lights should be dimmed, and outside noises should be minimized. Try to avoid interruptions. Breathe smoothly and rhythmically, allowing your body to release tension and relax. Then imagine a scene of your own choosing, trying to make the image as vivid and real as possible. This scene can be used therapeutically to help you feel better.

Walter was experiencing a sharp pain in his pelvic area. He was instructed to relax and then develop an image of what this pain looked like. He imagined it as a very sharp knife being jabbed into the area. Walter was then instructed to slowly reverse the action he had pictured. So Walter imagined the knife slowly being removed from his pelvis, and a soothing, healing cream being applied. Finally, the knife was completely out. Walter was then able to deepen his relaxation, greatly reducing his discomfort.

There are other images you could use to reduce pain. For example, you could initially imagine your bones being hit by a hammer or stuck with dozens of pins. Then, to reverse the image, you could imagine the hammer or pins being removed. Or you might think of cool air being blown across the affected area, or of the area being surrounded by warm water in a bathtub. Imagery is restricted only by your creativity, and can be used anywhere. (Have you ever taken a bath on a bus?!) Two good books on the subject are *In the Mind's Eye* by Arnold Lazarus and *Visualization for Change* by Patrick Fanning. See if your public library or local bookstore has them.

Hypnosis

Hypnosis involves a calm repetition of words and statements designed to induce a state of deep relaxation in which there is a heightened receptivity to suggestion. During this state, verbal suggestions help the mind to block your awareness of pain and replace it with a more positive feeling. While hypnosis is often quite effective in the area of pain control, it does not work for everybody. Also, in some cases, it is not effective in dealing with severe pain.

You can learn how to hypnotize yourself so that this technique can be used whenever you need it. However, the technique must first be learned from a professional—a licensed psychologist or a certified hypnotherapist, for instance. Many good books on clinical hypnosis can give you further information about this valuable tool.

Biofeedback

Biofeedback combines the techniques of relaxation and imagery, already discussed, with the use of measuring instruments, usually electronic ones. These machines give you feedback in the form of sounds or images, letting you know what's going on inside your body. In fact, biofeedback provides moment-by-moment information about the effect that your imagery and relaxation techniques are having on your physiological responses. What responses can be measured? Most frequently, the biofeedback units measure skin temperature, pulse, blood pressure, the electrical activity resulting from muscular tension, or the electrical activity coming from the brain.

How exactly can biofeedback help you control pain? Electrodes connected to the biofeedback unit are taped or otherwise attached to your skin. These electrodes monitor one of the physiological responses mentioned above, and transmit the information they pick up to the biofeedback unit in the form of electrical impulses. The unit then translates this feedback into sounds, lights, or pictures that you can hear or observe. Using this information, you can experiment and find the types of imagery and other relaxation techniques that will allow you to best control your internal responses, and thus induce relaxation and reduce muscle pain.

Gary was experiencing a lot of pain in his left leg, so his physician suggested that he try biofeedback. A machine measuring muscle tension was attached to the area of the leg in which he was experiencing the pain, in much the same way that electrodes from an EKG machine are connected. (Don't worry. There is no pain, and you won't get jolted!) As Gary attempted to relax the area, the machine let him know if he was really relaxing and also how well he was relaxing. As he became aware of his lessening tension, Gary learned which mental images worked best for him. Eventually, he was able to use the imagery on his own, without the machine, to help control his pain.

Certified biofeedback professionals can be found throughout the country. Check with your physician or your local hospital or clinic for names of professionals in your area.

Psychological Coping Strategies

By now, you probably understand the connection between emotions and pain, and want to do everything you can to decrease your fear, stress, tension, and other negative emotions—emotions that may make you more aware of pain or even *increase* your pain. Chapters 9 through 16 should help you pinpoint the source of your emotional distress and then find ways of better coping with your feelings. If you haven't already read these chapters, now would be a great time to give them a try. Never underestimate the effect that emotions can have on your physical health!

Of course, the more time you have to think about your pain, the worse it will seem. So try to divert your attention. Develop interests that require concentration—model building, crossword puzzles, or whatever suits your fancy. You can always come up with activities and thoughts that will entertain your mind while increasing your feeling of physical well-being.

PAIN CONTROL RESOURCES

You can learn and gain access to many pain-control techniques from your own physician; from mental-health professionals, including psychologists who specialize in certain pain-control techniques; and from other health professionals. Or you may want to read some of the books on pain control that are available in bookstores and libraries. Certainly, many techniques can be used at home—although, in some cases, they may work better if you learn them from clinics or centers. In fact, certain clinics specialize in the control of pain.

You might also want to get involved in a support group for people living with pain. To find a group in your area, check with your physician or your local hospital. It can be comforting to know that you're not alone in trying to cope with pain. You may even learn some new pain-control strategies.

Despite the effectiveness of the many pain-control techniques available today, it's important to consult your physician to make sure that any or all of the techniques you're considering are appropriate for you, and will pose no danger to your health. And, of course, your physician may make you aware of further coping techniques, one of which might be just the ticket!

AN UNAGONIZING CONCLUSION

Unfortunately, you may experience some pain as a result of prostate cancer. But don't throw in the heating pad! Realize that the pain need not last forever. A lot can be done, both medically and psychologically, to increase your level of comfort and help you more fully enjoy each and every day.

Chapter 20

OTHER PHYSICAL SYMPTOMS AND SIDE EFFECTS

Any chronic medical condition can affect you both physically and psychologically. We've already discussed how you can better cope with your emotions and with the pain of prostate cancer. And we've looked at ways in which you can deal with some of the specific side effects of prostate cancer treatment—the skin problems associated with radiation therapy and the hot flashes that sometimes accompany hormone therapy, for instance. In this chapter, we'll look at other physical effects of prostate cancer and its treatment—problems that, as mentioned before, can play a major role in your psychological adjustment to prostate cancer.

Certainly, it is important to be aware of the symptoms you may experience as a result of the cancer itself. You may not have all—or any!—of them; you may not be able to do something about all the ones you do have. But a number of the symptoms can be controlled either medically or through self-management and lifestyle changes. Might there be physical symptoms that you can't do anything about? Unfortunately, yes. And in that case, you'll have to learn to simply accept them. This may seem like a tall order, but what choice do you have? Try to concentrate on the things you *can* do something about. Deal with the symptoms as they come, if and when they come. Don't anticipate the worst, because that won't help you. It's far better to put your energy into positive efforts.

The side effects of cancer treatment, just like the symptoms of the cancer itself, may or may not occur in your case. Certainly, there are many people who undergo treatment for cancer without experiencing any side effects at all. Still, in case side effects do become a problem, it's wise to be prepared—to know what to look for, and when you should speak to your doctor. Some side effects—like some symptoms—may simply have to be endured. In other cases, though, you will be able to control the side effects and make life more comfortable for yourself.

So let's discuss some of the common symptoms and side effects of prostate cancer and its treatments. When there's something you can do about them, suggestions will be offered. When no treatments or management techniques are available, you'll at least learn more about the symptoms and become aware that you're not alone in experiencing them.

FATIGUE

Do you become more tired more easily now? Is your bed your favorite place to be in the whole world? If so, you're definitely not alone. Fatigue (yawn!) is a very common and unpleasant problem of people with cancer. In fact, fatigue is one of the most common symptoms of virtually every medical disorder!

Fatigue may show up following some activity or expenditure of energy. Or, without having done anything tiring, your body may suddenly decide it needs a rest cure! You may feel like the energy has drained right out of your body, like water draining from a leaky radiator. You may awaken in the morning feeling fine, and then have fatigue hit you during the day. On the other hand, you may awaken in the morning feeling very tired, and find that your energy builds during the day.

Why does fatigue occur? Fatigue may, of course, be caused by the cancer itself. It may also be caused by cancer treatments—either by the treatment itself, or by a buildup of waste products caused by the treatment's destruction of cells. Radiation treatments, for instance, sap a tremendous amount of energy, often causing fatigue and weakness. Pain, too, may cause fatigue.

Sometimes, fatigue is totally unrelated to the cancer and its treatment. You may simply be doing too much! As discussed earlier in the book, emotions such as stress, anxiety, and depression may also contribute to fatigue. Or it may be caused or exacerbated by nutritional problems, such as an insufficient intake of calories.

Sometimes fatigue can snowball. If you're chronically tired, you may cut down on your day-to-day activities, and this may result in even more fatigue. Unless something happens to break this chain, you may have less and less energy.

Fatigue may also result from cutting down on exercise, either because you can't exercise or because you feel that you shouldn't exercise, as it might worsen your condition. Of course, exercise need not be harmful, and can often be quite helpful. But if you allow your fears to keep you inactive, you may quickly become out of shape. And, of course, the less you do, the more out of shape and fatigued you'll become!

Most people think of fatigue as negative, but this is not always the case.

Fatigue can be positive. How? Usually, fatigue is your body's way of telling you that you need rest. If you never felt tired, you would push yourself too much! So if you feel fatigued, discuss this with your doctor. Together, you'll be able to decide what most likely is causing your fatigue.

What Can You Do?

What's the best way to cope with fatigue? Usually, rest is the answer. (Clever!) Other strategies for dealing with fatigue depend on the nature and cause of the fatique, of course, but you should always make sure to get the proper amount of rest so that your body can nourish and heal itself.

Allow yourself longer periods of time for sleep at night, and try to arrange for at least one or two brief rest periods during the day, preferably in the late morning and late afternoon. Although this added rest may not make your fatigue disappear, it certainly will help. But remember that that too much rest can actually lead to more fatigue! So make sure that you're getting the proper amounts and types of exercise. Exercise helps to break the cycle of fatigue and out-of-shape conditioning. (See Chapter 22 for more about exercise.)

Fatigue can also be reduced by efficient planning and pacing. Figure out exactly what your responsibilities are, and schedule activities so that you won't do too many strenuous things in a row. (For more about prioritizing, see page 152.) And be flexible. Be ready to change course if fatigue hits you out of the blue, or if you have a sudden burst of energy!

In some cases, you may want to modify the activity itself. For example, perhaps you are an avid golfer, and you normally spend six hours a day on the links. This may not be possible—or appropriate!—now. But you may be able to play nine holes of golf instead of eighteen.

Certainly, at various periods during your treatment, you may be more fatigued than you are at other times. During some treatments—radiation, for instance—you may need to take time off from your normal schedule. Rest assured, though, that you'll be able to return to a more normal routine once treatment is over and your energy has been restored.

Be willing to ask for help. Have other people accomplish some of the tasks that are lower priorities for you or don't demand your personal attention. This will conserve your energy, allowing you to do those things that are more important.

Just as important as getting needed rest and pacing yourself is a proper diet with sufficient calories. Try to eat regular, well-balanced meals. Also speak to your doctor about supplements, as they can insure that you're getting the nutrients you need. (For more information on diet, see Chapter 21.)

Finally, consider that your fatigue may be caused or worsened by emotions. Try to determine which emotional reactions are contributing to your fatigue. (Are you depressed? Bored? Anxious?) Then work on improving your outlook. (Chapters 9 through 16 should help you pinpoint and control any emotional problems.)

SLEEP PROBLEMS

People with cancer may occasionally experience sleep problems. These problems, especially insomnia, may result from pain, frequent urination, nausea, or other symptoms and side effects. Emotions, also, may play havoc with your sleeping patterns. Depression, for example, often causes too much sleep, while anxiety often causes too little.

What Can You Do?

Obviously, if your sleep problems are rooted in emotional troubles, you should work on better coping with your emotions. And if certain symptoms or side effects are keeping you up at night, appropriate treatment may help you to get the rest you need.

But what if these tactics aren't appropriate or completely successful? Before retiring in the evening, try eating foods that are high in tryptophan, a naturally occurring chemical that promotes sleep. Tryptophan-high foods include turkey, bananas, figs, dates, yogurt, tuna, and nut butter. You've probably heard that having a glass of warm milk right before bedtime can help. Well, it can! And as long as we're talking about foods, try to avoid caffeine—coffee, tea, cola, and chocolate—and alcohol before going to bed. These substances, as well as cigarettes, are all stimulants, and are therefore incompatible with the relaxation you need to fall sleep.

Because many people with sleep problems are mentally tired but not physically tired, you might try to get some exercise in the early evening. Hopefully, this will get your physical fatigue to match your mental fatigue, easing you into dreamland.

Also try using relaxation techniques—especially a muscle-relaxing technique such as the Quick Release. These techniques can be successful not only before going to bed, but also during the night when you awaken and have difficulty getting back to sleep. (See Chapter 19 for a discussion of relaxation techniques.)

As much as possible, regularize your sleep-wake cycle by getting to sleep at about the same time each night, and getting up at about the same time every morning. This may help your body respond more effectively to bedtime routines. And try to stick to the same routine each night. For instance, every night at ten o'clock, you might drink a glass of milk, read in bed for twenty minutes, and then turn off the light.

Try to minimize the length of any daytime naps, especially those that occur late in the day. Short naps are okay, especially if you can't hold your head up, but don't let the naps drag on, or you might find the nights dragging on as well.

Finally, if you simply can't sleep, rest! Research has shown that rest does provide some very important "recharging" benefits, and may also take some of the pressure off of you. What pressure? Why, the pressure to sleep, of course! And the pressure to sleep can keep you awake!

URINARY INCONTINENCE

Urinary incontinence—the inability to control urination—is a common problem of people with prostate cancer. This condition may be either temporary or permanent, depending on the severity of the prostate cancer as well as the treatment that you're undergoing. For instance, during a radical prostatectomy, the sphincter muscles that control urination may be damaged—although recent improvements in surgery have decreased the chance of this happening. Urinary incontinence may also result from the spread of prostate cancer to the pelvic region, where tumors can press on the bladder, causing a quicker release of urine.

What Can You Do?

Because incontinence is not as isolated a problem as you might expect, a number of excellent products are available to help you deal with incontinence in a way that minimizes the chance of accidents occurring. For example, mini pads, maxi pads, and adult diapers can all help prevent accidents. Or a device called the Cunningham clamp can be placed on the penis to stop leakage. Another device, the Maguire urinal, is worn much as an athletic supporter is worn, and includes a little pouch that drains urine into a leg bag.

Of course, any incontinence problems should be reported to your urologist. Then, once the source of the problem has been discovered, an appropriate treatment may be prescribed. For example, either medication or surgery may be used to lessen sphincter problems, as well as other conditions that cause incontinence. Special exercises such as Kegels, psychological techniques such as biofeedback, and other treatments have also been successful in reversing or controlling this condition.

When urinary incontinence has continued untreated, it is sometimes necessary to use self-induced catheterization in order to maintain urinary control. In this case, you will be taught to place a catheter—a small, flexible tube—in the bladder through the penis, enabling drainage of urine into a collection pouch.

Remember that although urinary incontinence is certainly inconvenient, it does not have to interfere at all with your way of life. With appropriate treatment and management techniques, you can continue enjoying all your usual activities.

DIARRHEA

Diarrhea—characterized by frequent, loose stools and painful stomach cramps—can be either a symptom of cancer or a side effect of cancer treatment. Most commonly, it is the result of radiation therapy.

What Can You Do?

Often, diarrhea can be reduced or eliminated with dietary changes, such as high-calorie, high-protein diets that are low in fat, fiber, coffee, and spices. Medication can also be helpful, especially if the diarrhea persists for prolonged periods of time. Many radiation therapists, for instance, suggest taking the over-the-counter product Pepto-Bismol. If this doesn't help, prescription drugs such as Lomotil may be effective. As long as the diarrhea remains a problem, fluids should be increased to prevent dehydration.

NAUSEA AND VOMITING

Nausea and vomiting, like diarrhea, can be caused either by the cancer itself or by the treatment.

What Can You Do?

If you are suffering from nausea, you may find that salty foods are easiest to get down, and that cold foods—which usually have less of an odor than hot foods do—are also relatively palatable. Certainly, you'll want to avoid strong-smelling, greasy foods. And since food odors may nauseate you even in the absence of the foods themselves, you'll probably want to stay away from places in which food is being prepared.

You may be tempted to ask for your favorite foods, thinking that these will be most appealing. Be aware, though, that this isn't always the wisest strategy during bouts of nausea. Why? After the nausea diminishes, you may find yourself turned off by your former favorites!

Family members or friends may suggest that you drink carbonated beverages in order to reduce your feelings of nausea. Yes, this can help, but be aware that this technique is most helpful when the beverage is allowed to stand for a while and "flatten."

If your nausea continues, your physician may prescribe an antinausea medication such as Compazine (prochlorperazine).

LOSS OF APPETITE

Loss of appetite, due to either the cancer itself or treatments, is a very common problem for people with prostate cancer. This may occur for any of a number of reasons, including changes in your ability to taste, nausea, and stress or other psychological factors.

What Can You Do?

If your appetite has been reduced, try to eat small, frequent meals rather than larger meals, which may prove intimidating. If loss of appetite has been troubling you for some time, you may need to take supplements that will help stabilize you nutritionally. And, of course, your treatment should be aimed at reducing the symptoms of cancer that may be affecting your appetite. Finally, if you feel that your emotions are partly responsible for your loss of appetite, the appropriate coping strategies may help to restore your appetite.

A PHYSICAL FINALE

This chapter has discussed a number of the physical symptoms and side effects that may occur because of prostate cancer or its treatment. Although these physical effects are not pleasant to think about, it's important to find out as much about them as you can. You want to learn how to cope with prostate cancer, right? By marshalling all your forces to control these problems, you'll not only improve your level of comfort, but also build the confidence you need to continue leading a strong, productive life.

Chapter 21

DIET

Are you eating less and enjoying it less? Research has shown that cancer, as well as its treatment, can affect your eating habits, and, accordingly, your weight. In addition, more and more research is now focusing on connections between diet and cancer. Therefore, it makes sense that any person who has prostate cancer should work to control his eating patterns, and try to follow as healthy a diet as possible.

Why is nutrition so important, and what exactly *is* a good diet? Let's learn more about diet and prostate cancer, and see what you can do to maximize your health.

WHY IS NUTRITION SO IMPORTANT?

Nutrition is the process of taking in appropriate amounts of nutrients and using them to meet energy needs, to accomplish body-sustaining healing, and to satisfy maintenance requirements. Here are just some of the benefits a sound diet may provide for the person with prostate cancer:

- ☐ A body that is well nourished is stronger than a poorly nourished body is. So proper nourishment enables the body to better fight infection, aids healing, and promotes well-being.
- ☐ A good diet actually helps individuals respond better to prostate cancer treatment, and makes them more resistant to treatment side effects.
- ☐ Good nutrition provides good energy. Everybody needs fuel to energize the body. And because of the potential energy-zapping effects of prostate cancer treatments—and of the cancer itself— proper diet is doubly important for men with prostate cancer.
- ☐ Body tissues may break down as a result of aggressive prostate cancer treatment. A balanced diet increases the speed at which body tissues heal themselves, and helps prevent them from breaking down in the first place.

☐ Without proper nutrition, the body's stores of protein, vitamins, and other nutrients may be depleted in unhealthy ways. A good diet insures continuing healthy stores of these nutrients.

☐ A sound diet limits fat, which appears to be linked to the development of prostate cancer. Therefore, a good diet may actually help keep cancer in check.

☐ A sound diet—which, according to current dietary guidelines, is rich in fresh fruits and vegetables—provides cancer-protective nutrients.

DIETARY RECOMMENDATIONS

As discussed in Chapter 2, some experts believe that the different rates of prostate cancer in different parts of the world imply an environmental basis, in which case, nutrition may play an important part in determining which cultures have higher or lower incidences of the disorder. Certainly, studies indicate that there is, in fact, a link between diet and cancer. At this time, there is no specific "prostate cancer cure diet," although there are many good books describing the role of nutrition in cancer prevention and treatment. However, there are some important dietary recommendations for individuals with prostate cancer.

Perhaps it's best to begin our discussion by briefly looking at the United States Department of Agriculture's (USDA's) most current dietary recommendations. If, like most of us, you remember the "four basic food groups," which heavily emphasized the importance of meat, poultry, and dairy, the new guidelines may prove startling. Basing their recommendations on current research—including cancer studies—the USDA now recommends a complex-carbohydrate, low-fat, high-fiber diet. The government has made it clear that whole grains, fruits, and vegetables should form the base of a good diet. Of lesser importance are the dairy group and the meat, poultry, and fish group. Fats, oils, and sweets, the government states, should be used only sparingly.

Certainly, the USDA guidelines make good sense for the person with prostate cancer. But let's take a closer look at some specific recommendations for the person who's learning to cope with this disorder.

Eat a Low-Fat Diet

One of the reasons that cancer rates are different in different parts of the world may be the amount of fat consumed in different cultures. Studies of prostate cancer mortality rates in a number of countries suggest that more prostate cancer deaths occur in countries in which high-fat diets are prevalent—countries like the United States. And a study released by the Harvard School of Public Health in 1993—just one of several studies with similar findings—states that people who eat red meat five times a week are 2.6 times more likely to develop advanced, often fatal prostate cancer, than are people who eat red meat once a week or less.

How do fats—especially animal fats—promote prostate cancer? While scientists aren't sure, several theories have been offered to explain this phenomenon. Possibly, animal fats alter sex hormone levels in the blood. (As you know, higher levels of these hormones lead to the growth of prostate cancer.) Or carcinogens—cancer-producing agents—may be formed when animal fat is cooked. Or the fatty acids found in meat may interfere with cell function.

Whatever the link may be between fat consumption and prostate cancer, clearly, it is wise to reduce your fat intake—especially since cutting down on dietary fat also reduces the risk of heart disease and many other disorders. Most important is the reduction of animal fats, as these seem to be most strongly linked to prostate cancer. How, exactly, can you reduce the fat in your diet? Limit your consumption of red meat to about once every ten days, and eat only lean red meat. Eat more white-meat poultry and fish, excluding shellfish, sardines, mackerel, and fish canned in oil, all of which are high in fat and cholesterol. Limit your consumption of dairy products, and eat only nonfat dairy products. Also limit yourself to only a few egg whites—or the equivalent amount of a cholesterol-free egg substitute—a week. And, as far as possible, eliminate oils and fats, including butter, margarine, lard, and vegetable oils. When oils can't be totally avoided, stick to polyunsaturated oils, such as olive, peanut, canola, and safflower.

Eat a High-Fiber Diet

Many studies have indicated that low-fiber diets are major contributors to the risk of cancer. High-fiber diets, on the other hand, seem to lower the risk of cancer. How does fiber protect us? Fiber—the part of plant materials that our body does not digest—binds bile acids, cholesterol, carcinogens, and other substances that lead to cancer. Fiber also increases the weight and amount of stool, which eliminates carcinogens.

Fortunately, it's easy—and delicious—to add more fiber to your diet. High-fiber cereals are the best source of this important nutrient. Also good are vegetables such as Brussels sprouts, broccoli, and cabbage—which, as you'll learn later in the chapter, are also an excellent source of certain cancer-protective agents. Whole-grain breads, pasta, and whole or lightly milled grains like rice, barley, and buckwheat are other good sources of fiber.

Eat a Diet High in Antioxidants

While proper levels of all vitamins and minerals are necessary for normal body functions, certain vitamins have been found to be particularly helpful in the fight against cancer. Vitamins A, C, and E—as well as beta-carotene, the chemical used by the body to make vitamin A—and the mineral selenium help the body protect itself. Known as *antioxidants*, these nutrients block the cancer-initiation process and help preserve the cell's DNA, the genetic material necessary for healthy cell reproduction. A sufficient amount of these nutrients as part of a well-balanced diet can help prevent cancer, can help fight cancer, and can help prevent the recurrence of cancer.

What foods are richest in these cancer-protective nutrients? Active vitamin A is found only in animal sources, such as cod liver oil, beef, and chicken. However, beta-carotene, the vitamin A precursor, is found in green and yellow-orange vegetables and fruits, including carrots, kale, kohlrabi, spinach, turnip greens, dandelion greens, apricots, and cantaloupe. Some of the foods highest in vitamin C are broccoli, Brussels sprouts, kale, turnip greens, parsley, sweet peppers, cabbage, cauliflower, and spinach. Vitamin E is found in vegetable oils, such as corn, soybean, and safflower oil, and in whole grains, dark green leafy vegetables, nuts, and legumes. Selenium is found mostly in seafoods and whole grains.

Clearly, a diet high in fresh fruits and vegetables and whole grains is likely to be high in the nutrients known to be cancer-fighters. And some of these foods may have protective elements above and beyond the vitamins discussed above. For instance, studies indicate that broccoli contains a substance that helps to guard against tumor formation. In fact, the American Cancer Society has urged us to eat more vegetables from the cruciferous group—which includes broccoli, cabbage, Brussels sprouts, and cauliflower—as this group seems to have cancer-preventive properties.

One final note. When adding fruits and vegetables to your diet, be sure to get the freshest produce possible, as it will have the highest levels of nutrients. If possible, eat the vegetables raw, as heat can destroy nutrients. When cooking vegetables, steam or microwave them briefly to preserve nutrient content.

Avoid Harmful "Nonfoods"

In addition to some of the foods you may be eating, a number of nonfoods—additives, pesticides, caffeine, alcohol, and tobacco—can also contribute to cancer. Let's take a brief look at each of the nonfoods that may now be in your diet.

Artificial Additives

Believe it or not, the average American diet includes 5,000 or more artificial additives each year. These additives are used to maintain freshness, preserve the attractive look or taste of food, or help in the preparation of food. While some of these additives are safe, many have been linked to cancer or are suspected as being cancer initiators, while others have not undergone sufficient studies to determine their safety.

What can you do to eliminate all—or, at least, many—of these additives from your diet? Obviously, additives are most common in processed foods—canned foods, frozen foods, and prepared foods of all kinds. Avoid these foods whenever you can. Instead, eat whole foods that are as close as possible to their natural state. When you do buy prepared foods, choose those that have been made without additives. And avoid smoked foods, which contain some of the most harmful additives used in food processing.

Pesticides

Like additives, pesticides, used to control weeds and pests, are abundant in your diet. In fact, unless you eat only organic food that has been grown in pesticide-free soil, you consume pesticides every day in meat, poultry, fish, dairy products, vegetables, fruits, coffee—virtually all your foods. Many of these pesticides—some of which are banned in the United States, but reach us through produce from other countries—are known or suspected to be associated with cancer.

How can you avoid pesticides? Scrub or peel all fruits and vegetables, and always peel waxed fruit. If possible, buy organically grown foods, and avoid imported produce, which may contain banned chemicals. Finally, be aware that a diet high in fiber and antioxidants can help eliminate pesticides from your body.

Alcohol

Excessive alcohol consumption has been linked to an increased risk of a number of cancers. In addition, alcohol is known to be so damaging to the immune system that some consider it a strong immune-suppressive drug.

Is it necessary to avoid all alcohol? There's no simple answer to this question. However, it seems wise to reduce your consumption of alcohol as much as possible. One drink a week is considered a safe amount. Less is better. After all, you want to do all you can do make your body strong and healthy!

Caffeine

Like alcohol, caffeine—found in coffee, tea, colas, chocolate, and other foods—has been linked to several types of cancer. It is also known that caffeine can cause damage to DNA, potentially leading to the development of cancer.

Again, if you want to do everything possible to build yourself up, it makes sense to avoid caffeine. And what should take the place of your coffee, tea, and caffeinated beverages? Your best bets are skim milk, mineral water, unsweetened fruit juices, and vegetable juices. Besides eliminating harmful caffeine, most of these drinks take a further step toward improving your health by supplying valuable nutrients.

Tobacco

Finally, we come to tobacco. By now, most of us know that tobacco smoke has been implicated in several cancers. Smoking also causes great damage to the immune system. And chewing tobacco and snuff have been found to be just as harmful as smoking tobacco.

In the case of tobacco, the best course of action is clear. By avoiding all tobacco—including other people's smoke—you'll strengthen your body against not only cancer, but also a number of other diseases.

GETTING STARTED

Now you know why a good diet is such an important part of your program of treatment, and you also have learned a little about current general dietary recommendations and about specific recommendations for people with cancer. Certainly, regardless of what stage your prostate cancer is in, you can make your body better able to fight the disease. So it's time to get started—to make the changes necessary to create the healthiest diet possible! Here are a few suggestions.

☐ To begin modifying your diet, keep a food diary by writing down everything you eat. This will give you a realistic look at your present diet, and will suggest ways in which you can make improvements.

☐ Decrease the fat in your diet by limiting your consumption of meat, and increasing your consumption of fresh fruits and vegetables and whole grains.

☐ Decrease your consumption of dairy foods, and make sure that the dairy foods you do eat are nonfat.

☐ Eat all foods in a form as close as possible to their natural state. This will maximize their vitamins, minerals, and fiber, and minimize additives.

☐ When possible, eat organically grown produce. When this isn't available, be sure to scrub or peel fruits and vegetables to eliminate pesticides. Always peel waxed produce.

☐ Do what you can to avoid harmful nonfoods—additives, pesticides, alcohol, caffeine, and tobacco. While you may not be able to avoid all of these substances all of the time, by cutting them down as far as possible, you'll be doing a great deal to improve your overall health.

☐ Avoid "empty" calories. Cookies, potato chips, and candy, for instance, have little or no nutritional value, and may keep you from eating vitamin- and fiber-rich foods. In addition, many of these foods are laden with fat, a known risk factor in cancer.

☐ To help insure an adequate intake of vitamins and minerals—especially the antioxidants—consider including vitamin and mineral supplements in your dietary program. Speak to your doctor about the supplements that will be best for you.

☐ Eat regularly. If digestion occurs on a regular and frequent basis, your blood sugars will be kept from fluctuating wildly, and you'll enjoy greater energy and fewer mood swings. Frequent smaller meals may be the answer.

☐ Include physical activity in your dietary program. Besides toning your body, exercise before a meal can stimulate your appetite. (See Chapter 22 for more about exercise.)

☐ If you're suffering from nausea or loss of appetite, try frequent smaller meals. (See Chapter 20 for more tips on fighting nausea.)

☐ Consider the fact that your appetite may vary based on how you feel on any given day. During times when you're feeling better, make sure that you eat all the nutrient-packed foods you can to compensate for those times when you feel less well.

☐ Stay informed! The more you know about the link between diet and cancer, the better able you'll be to make healthy, cancer-fighting dietary changes. To begin, you might try reading Dr. Charles Simone's *Cancer and Nutrition*, a comprehensive book designed to help you create your own anticancer diet.

Before modifying your diet, be sure to speak to your physician. He or she will be able to guide you in making the modifications that are right for you. Also keep in mind that although proper diet is an important part of any treatment program—and is almost totally within the control of the individual—it is also one of the most frequently ignored means of treatment. While it may be difficult for you to change your eating habits, once you begin to eliminate any harmful foods and to increase your intake of nutrient-rich foods, you're sure to feel healthier and more energetic. And you'll benefit from the peace of mind that comes from doing everything you can to help yourself. So eat healthy, eat wisely, and enjoy!

Chapter 22

EXERCISE

In Chapter 20, you learned how extra rest can help you cope with fatigue and give your body a chance to heal and "recharge." But you also learned that too much rest can make you feel more tired, leading to more rest, more fatigue, more rest. . . . You get the picture! What's the solution? Exercise! The right types and amounts of exercise can help you break the fatigue-rest-fatigue cycle and make you feel better in countless other ways. In this chapter, you'll learn about the many benefits of exercise, and see how you—with the help of your physician—can design your own personal exercise program.

THE BENEFITS OF EXERCISE

Exercise is important for everyone, but is especially important for those with a medical problem such as prostate cancer. Why? Exercise can be helpful in keeping your body trim. And for best health, you should keep your muscles firm, firm, firm, which is better than flabby, flabby, flabby. Exercise can also help your body systems—including your cardiovascular and digestive systems—work more efficiently. As a result, a person who participates in regular exercise usually has more energy, has fewer physical complaints, and sleeps better than a more sedentary person. Is that all? Nope! Exercise can also reduce pain and make you feel less fatigued. Exercise can even increase your appetite.

And exercise is as good for your psychological well-being as it is for your body. Have you lost some self-esteem as a result of your condition? Exercise can restore some of your self-confidence and make you feel more capable—more in control. Living with prostate cancer may have also increased your level of stress. Exercise is a great release for that stress! (For many people, exercise is more calming than a tranquilizer, and has no side effects.) Through exercise, you can let off steam, relieve any boredom and frustration, and clear your mind. In fact, all of the emotions that may be troubling you—depression, anger, and anxiety among them—can be controlled, either wholly or partly, through exercise. And if that's not enough of a lure, unless you exercise alone, your exercise program will lead to some healthy social interactions—which are always good for the mind!

SO, WHY AREN'T YOU EXERCISING?

Considering all the good things that exercise does, you may wonder why everybody isn't out there working out. Well, many people feel that exercise is, at best, boring, and, at worst, unpleasant. Only a small percentage of people really and truly enjoy regular exercise. (Are you one of them?) So the best approach is to focus on exercises—and exercise environments—that are as pleasant as possible! This will enable you to more easily keep your commitment to regular exercise.

Then again, some people may avoid exercise not because of a lack of desire, but because they find it so tiring. Or perhaps they fear that exercise may cause additional problems. While these feelings of fear and fatigue are understandable, as we've mentioned before, as you become less and less active, you will only *increase* your feelings of fatigue. Why? Because of deconditioning. Deconditioning—the result of inactivity—causes your muscles to grow weaker and weaker over time, giving you less and less energy. What are the symptoms of deconditioning? Shortness of breath, rapid heartbeat, and increased fatigue are the most common signs that deconditioning has taken place.

Guess what? Deconditioning can gradually be reduced. How? Through exercise! By embarking on a gradually building exercise program, you can slowly increase your ability to participate in these activities. How can you begin? Stay tuned!

GETTING STARTED

Before beginning any exercise program, you should, of course, consult with your physician. Once your physician has okayed your program, you must commit yourself to it. There is no benefit to be gained by exercising for a day or two, and then giving up. If you want to feel better, you'll have to exercise regularly. But be patient. Most exercise programs really don't show results for three or four weeks, if not more. As long as you stick to your exercise program, though, you *will* see results.

Anybody who attempts to accelerate an exercise program to bring about faster results will end up suffering—and, possibly, abandoning the program. So implement your exercise program gradually. In fact, the longer it's been since you've done any exercising, the slower your return should be.

Expect the first few weeks of your program to be the most difficult. Why? Because if you haven't been very active lately, you're probably out of shape. This is not meant as a put-down. Your muscles simply need time to regain their strength. So expect increased fatigue for a while, as well as a few new aches and pains. These temporary discomforts are perfectly normal, and will disappear as you consistently participate in a gradual exercise program.

How often must you exercise in order to reap the benefits of physical activity? Usually, you must exercise three or four times a week, for a minimum of twenty minutes each time, in order to recondition your body. However, some people have found that they feel best when they exercise five or six times a week. Gradually, you'll find out what works for you.

EXERCISING CAUTION

We've already mentioned the importance of working with a physician or other health-care professional when starting an exercise program. This will not just insure that the program you've chosen is safe, but will also give you a "partner" in your program—someone who will help you keep track of what you're doing and how it's helping you. If you're working with a health spa or club, you should, of course, inform the staff of your condition. But remember that they are not experts in prostate cancer! So be sure to okay any exercise program recommended by the club with your doctor.

It's also vital to make sure that when you exercise, you do it properly, following appropriate guidelines and safety rules. Again, do not build up your pace too quickly. You'll want to follow a concept in exercise known as the "progression principle." This principle states that exercise should be started slowly, and, as time goes by, increased in intensity.

Earlier we mentioned that you should expect to feel more aches and pains as you begin your program. But it's important to learn the difference between muscle soreness, which is probably a normal response to exercise, and acute pain. Acute pain may mean that you're overdoing it, or that you're participating in an exercise that's a no-no. The old saying "No pain, no gain" is not true when you have a medical problem. So if the discomfort you feel is extreme, by all means, stop exercising, and consult with a professional. You may have to choose a different form of exercise or to otherwise modify your routine.

CATEGORIES OF EXERCISES

While all exercises can be used to improve stamina and muscle tone, different types have other aims, as well. It is these other goals that determine the category into which a particular exercise falls. How many categories are there? Most exercises belong in one of four groups: muscle-stretching exercises, aerobic exercises, muscle-strengthening exercises, and range-of-motion exercises. Which types should you choose? Well, it's usually important to include exercises that will maintain muscle tone, normal joint motion, and overall fitness. So you'll probably want to incorporate a few different types of exercises—muscle-stretching and aerobics, for example—into your program. Of course, your choice will depend partly on your own specific needs, and partly on your own preferences.

Once you've chosen the exercises for your program, you'll want to make sure to perform these exercises in a particular order each time you do your routine. Most routines, you see, begin with a warm-up, which uses stretching exercises to ready you for more vigorous activity; proceed to the main part of the routine—the aerobics, for instance; and end with a cool-down period. This sequence helps prevent injury, and leaves you feeling exhilarated at the end of the routine.

Let's look at the four categories of exercise, and see what each type can do for you. Remember, though, that more important than the type of exercise you do is the regularity with which you perform your exercise routine. Consistency and persistence are the keys to improving your strength, endurance, flexibility, and general well-being.

Stretching Exercises

When joints are not being properly used due to inactivity, muscle cramping and inflexibility can result. In fact, when joints are stiff, even the smallest motion can cause pain. Stretching exercises help to eliminate any stiffness or tightness in the muscles, tendons, and ligaments surrounding the joints, relieving pain and preventing injury. As already mentioned, stretching exercises are a great way to begin any exercise routine. And, of course, they're beneficial exercises in and of themselves.

Where can you learn stretching exercises? If you belong to an exercise club, the instructors will certainly be able to show you some gentle, effective stretching exercises. And, of course, numerous exercise books and videotapes are available for all levels of proficiency.

Aerobic Exercises

By definition, an aerobic exercise is one that involves or improves oxygen consumption by requiring increased amounts of oxygen for prolonged periods of time. Doing aerobics for at least twenty minutes, a minimum of three times a week, can strengthen your heart, improve circulation, reduce blood pressure, and relieve tension. So aerobics can give you more energy, improve your endurance, and make you feel a whole lot happier, too.

As mentioned above, experts usually say that aerobics should be maintained for at least twenty minutes during each session. However, when you begin your exercise program, be careful not to overdo. Depending on your current level of fitness, consider starting with a sustained five- or ten-minute effort and gradually increasing the time as you feel stronger and have more confidence.

What are some examples of aerobic activities? Aerobics include brisk walking, jogging, riding a regular or stationary bicycle, climbing stairs, using a treadmill, aerobic dancing, and swimming. So, you see, you don't have to belong to a gym or buy a videotape to enjoy aerobics!

Are aerobics for you? Certainly, everybody can benefit from the many advantages aerobics have to offer. And aerobics are a good complement to stretching, range-of-motion, and muscle-strengthening exercises.

Muscle-Strengthening Exercises

Strengthening exercises are used to increase the size, and therefore the strength, of your muscles. For instance, isometrics, one type of muscle-strengthening exercise, work by pushing one immovable force against another. Trying to pull your hands apart after clasping them firmly, or pushing the palm of one hand against the palm of the other, are both isometrics. Isometric exercises are convenient in that they can be done anywhere—in the car, in a chair, even in bed. And although you won't be moving around, you'll still give your muscles a great workout.

Of course, isometrics aren't the only exercises in this category. Push-ups, sit-ups, and chin-ups—exercises you're probably quite familiar with—will also strengthen your muscles.

Where can you learn some appropriate muscle-strengthening exercises? Again, libraries, bookstores, videotape stores, and your local gym are likely to be your best resource.

Range-of-Motion Exercises

A range-of-motion exercise helps maintain or increase a joint's complete movement by moving a body part as far as possible in every direction. Moving a leg in large circles is one example of a range-of-motion exercise.

Like all other exercises, range-of-motion routines can be learned through books and videotapes, or from the staff of your local gym. Physical therapists can also help you out with this category of exercise.

GENERAL EXERCISE GUIDELINES

To make sure you derive the greatest benefits from your exercise program—without straining your muscles or worsening your symptoms—certain guidelines should be kept in mind. Some of the following points have not yet been mentioned in this chapter. Others have already been discussed, but are important enough to bear repeating.

☐ Don't feel that you have to wait until your prostate-cancer symptoms disappear before starting an exercise program! Involve yourself in exercises that will help you feel better *now*.

☐ Make sure you check with your physician before starting *any* exercise program. This way, you'll be sure that the program is right for you.

☐ Begin every exercise routine with a short warm-up. The best warm-ups use stretching exercises to limber the muscles, preparing the body for the more strenuous activities to follow.

☐ Develop your ability to tolerate exercise slowly. Certainly, one of your goals is to improve your strength and endurance, so you'll have to increase the length of time or intensity of your routine; but remember to do this gradually. Too rapid an increase, or too intense a program, may only worsen the pain that you're experiencing—as well as lessen your desire to exercise.

☐ Anticipate minor discomforts during your first days or weeks of exercising. Remember that you're doing things your body may not be used to doing! Some people feel it's a good idea to push yourself just a little (very little) beyond the point at which pain first occurs. This may help to increase your tolerance. But be careful. If the pain or discomfort seems excessive or lasts too long, be sure to tell your doctor. Probably, you're overdoing. Always listen to your body!

☐ Try to participate in activities that improve muscle tone, rather than building muscle bulk. For example, walking and swimming are far better than weight lifting!

☐ Rather than exercising whenever the spirit moves you, set aside a regular time each day or several days a week for your exercise routine. Then stick to your schedule!

☐ Don't compare your exercise program with somebody else's. You wouldn't compare your medication prescriptions with someone else's, would you? Remember that your situation—your special needs and limits—is unique.

☐ Initially, commit yourself to your exercise program for at least two months. By that time, you will probably be able to see the benefits of the program, and will be motivated to continue. This will decrease the chance of your becoming an exercise dropout.

☐ If you decide to join a gym for your exercise program, be on guard against instructors who tell you that they know "just what will make you feel better." They may know very little, if anything, about prostate cancer. On the other hand, they don't *need* to know much about prostate cancer—not as long as you check all of their suggestions with your doctor.

A FINAL EXERCISE

Exercise can be either extremely valuable or extremely harmful—or anything in between—depending on the care you use in choosing and following your program. Because every person is different, there is no one set of exercises that can be recommended for everyone. But everybody is capable of doing some exercises, and everybody can benefit from them. Just don't jump in feet first! Use your head. Speak to your physician—or, perhaps, to a physical therapist who's in touch with your physician. Then start slowly, build up your stamina, and enjoy your improved health!

Chapter 23

ACTIVITIES

What to do, what to do? Sure you have prostate cancer, but what does this mean in terms of the basic activities in your life? What can you do, and what can't you do? Even if you feel fine, you may be nervous about participating in any vigorous activities. You may want to minimize the strain you put on your body. Then again, you may not have the strength to even consider engaging in your usual activities!

Each person is different. The kinds of things you did before being diagnosed with prostate cancer will influence what you can or want to do now. Your current physical condition is also an important factor. If you're in the middle of treatment, you may not want to expend a lot of energy until your doctor has given you the green light—or even a cautious yellow—to resume. So let's discuss some of the activities that may concern you, and see how you can make various kinds of changes that will enable you to be as active as you want to be.

WORKING

Work helps you to feel independent. It gives you a sense of self-fulfillment and self-worth. It provides more financial strength than not working, of course. And it provides an important component of your social life. Understandably, you are probably quite concerned that your prostate cancer may interfere with your work. Perhaps you feel too tired to shoulder your usual workload. Or perhaps you feel fine, but you fear that your boss will assume that because you have prostate cancer, you can no longer do a good job. Let's look at some specific job-related concerns, and learn a little bit more about the ways in which prostate cancer can affect your work, and what you can do about it.

Should You Continue Working?

While some people with prostate cancer are eager to remain on the job, others question whether or not they *should* work. What's the answer? If you want to, you need to, and you can, then you should! Of course, you may have to make some modifications to avoid wearing yourself down. And, as you might suspect, it would be best to consult your doctor about any limitations that might be appropriate.

What If Fatigue or Other Discomforts Are a Problem?

You may be concerned that symptoms or side effects will prevent you from adequately performing on the job. Certainly, prostate cancer may cause you to experience fatigue and other discomforts, and this may affect your productivity—especially if your treatment is not controlling your symptoms as well as you'd like it to. You may get tired easily, and feel that you just don't have the stamina necessary to complete your job satisfactorily. Your work rate may have slowed down, and you may be absent or late more than usual. If your employer is aware of any of these problems, you may be afraid that your value to the company will be questioned—that your job may be in jeopardy.

What should you do? Pace yourself. Take rest breaks whenever necessary—and possible—to "recharge your batteries." If you've recently had surgery or other debilitating treatments, build your stamina up slowly. Don't expect too much all at once. And, of course, try to get more rest in the evenings. If you're not sure how much you can do, do what you can, and let your body be your guide.

What should you do if you find that you may have to shorten your hours or modify your work in some way? Well, you should be aware that employers are not required by law to make any special provisions for you because you have prostate cancer. You still have to do what you're supposed to do. However, if you're a valued employee, your company will probably be willing to make any minor modifications necessary to retain your services.

Of course, you may feel uncomfortable about approaching your employer to find out if any changes can be made in your work schedule or the work itself. It may bother you to seek "special treatment." Consider that any necessary modifications may be small in comparison to the ones your company would face if they had to hire a new employee to replace you!

Darius had been working in the same office for eighteen years. Lately, though, because of prostate cancer, he had been having more difficulty completing his responsibilities and getting to work on time. Unfortunately, his supervisor was a perfectionist who apparently was not willing to bend at all for Darius. He called him in for review and made it perfectly clear that unless his performance and attendance improved, he would be out of a job. As if that wasn't bad enough, the supervisor frequently reminded Darius that he was watching him. The pressure on Darius became so hard to bear that it began to affect his emotional and physical health.

What if your employer refuses to bend the rules? What if an ultimatum is given, stating that if productivity does not improve, you will be discharged? If this happens, simply do the best you can. If your employer doesn't understand enough about prostate cancer to know that you must pace yourself, and shows little or no willingness to cooperate, then you're probably better off not continuing employment there. You don't want to look for more trouble.

What if another employee resents any special treatment you've been given? Try to sit down, one-to-one, and have a conversation with your unhappy colleague. Explain your situation as much as necessary. Often, this is all that's needed to bring about greater understanding and cooperation. If your co-worker still doesn't understand, content yourself with knowing that you tried. Now it's his problem! (For more information on dealing with colleagues, see Chapter 28.)

Should You Discuss Your Condition With Your Employer?

How appropriate is it to discuss your medical condition itself with your employer? Obviously, there are some employers who will be very supportive and understanding, and there are others who will be somewhat apprehensive about retaining—or hiring—an individual who has any kind of cancer. Keep in mind that despite your employer's sympathy, he or she has a primary responsibility: keeping productivity at its highest possible level. So it may be helpful to reassure your employer that you'll work to keep your condition from interfering with your own productivity. The reality is that most people with prostate cancer can fulfill work obligations much the way anybody else can! If, at some point, modifications do have to be made, you'll deal with them—and your employer—at that time.

What If Employers Refuse to Retain or Hire You?

Employers may be hesitant to retain or hire someone with cancer for a number of reasons. For instance, an employer may feel that his or her health insurance premiums will be that much higher if you are listed on the plan, or even that the insurance carrier will cancel the existing coverage. Don't accept this argument sitting down. The Federal Rehabilitation Act of 1973 clearly states that it is against the law for anyone to refuse you appropriate work because you have cancer. (The act applies to many other medical conditions, as well.) So if you are denied a job or dismissed from your present job because of prostate cancer, don't take it sitting down. Instead, call the Equal Employment Opportunity Commission (EEOC). By dialing 800-669-4000, you'll be directed to the branch nearest you.

What About Returning to Work?

If you have completed treatment for prostate cancer, your return to work will be a very important step, not only for you, but for your family members, as well. For all concerned, the feeling will be that life is about to return to a more normal state of affairs.

If you've taken time off for surgery or other treatments, you may be worried that your return will not be as pleasant as you'd like. Co-workers may be very concerned about cancer, and may not react to you as they have in the past. Employers may fear that you will not be able to work as efficiently as you used to, or that you will need to take more time off because of ongoing treatments. Of course, it's possible that none of these problems will occur, but you may worry about them, nevertheless.

It may comfort you to know that the American Cancer Society has been working very hard to help individuals with cancer return to work comfortably, with a minimum of disruption. Through public education and legislation, problems affecting individuals who are returning to work will hopefully be reduced.

But what can you do now? Have confidence in yourself. The more positive your attitude and the better you present yourself, the more quickly any coolness on the part of others will disappear. Speak to those individuals who you feel are most receptive, and explain that you're perfectly capable of resuming your responsibilities. But remember that you can't change others. So strive to work on your own behavior and your own feelings.

What If You Have to Change Jobs?

Because of new limitations, your old job may no longer be right for you. If this is the case, you should certainly consider transferring to another job, even if it means getting additional training.

Lance, a fifty-nine-year-old father of two, had been working as a wall-paper hanger and handyman. But doctors felt that Lance shouldn't continue doing this type of work because it was too strenuous for him. Lance became very depressed. He didn't know what else he could do. He was afraid that any new training might be too difficult. Rather than face the prospect of being unable to work, Lance shut down emotionally. Fortunately, a good friend gave Lance an idea that allowed him to use his skills in another way. Lance hired and trained college students to do the actual wallpapering and repair work. In this way, he was able not only to continue to take jobs, but to actually expand his business—and without the undesirable physical exertion!

Certainly, the prospect of having to look for work is more daunting to some than it is to others. But if for any reason you are unable to continue working at your present job, don't despair. There are many ways in which you can get the training you need to move into a different type of position. Your first step might be to check with any of the government services that offer vocational counseling. Counselors in these offices will work with you to determine exactly what your aptitude is for different jobs. You will then be able to get the training and support you must have to obtain employment in the desired field. If you need help in finding jobs that are appropriate for you, your State Employment Services may be a good place to start. These services are available free of charge, and may guide you in locating jobs that will match your abilities and limitations. In addition, the Federal Rehabilitation Act of 1973 requires states to include all individuals with cancer in vocational rehabilitation programs to enable them to get back to work if their previous jobs are no longer appropriate for them. These programs vary from state to state, though, so it's important to check with your state's Office of Vocational Rehabilitation to find out what's available. Any financial adviser you're working with also should be able to help you in this regard.

Some people feel that for financial reasons, you should postpone looking for new employment until your old employment has been terminated. This tactic has its pros and cons. If you receive unemployment benefits for losing your job, this could ease your financial burden. But if subsequent employers are reluctant to hire you because of your grounds for dismissal, this tactic may explode in your face. Only you, with your unique knowledge of your own situation, can decide which course of action is right for you.

Is Working Your Only Option?

As you know, there are many benefits of working, including satisfaction, pride, and money. But a paying job is not the only type of satisfying work that's available. Many meaningful, productive activities can be pursued on a voluntary basis. Check with nonprofit charities, religious organizations, political groups, hospitals, schools, senior citizen centers, and the like. These organizations, and many more, can always use some extra help. Volunteer work may even allow you to explore an area of interest that you've never been able to participate in due to work commitments. And this work will help you feel good about yourself in the bargain.

What if you just don't want to work? If this is your preference, and you're able to manage without a job, that's great. But don't use your condition as an excuse for not working. Instead, try to find out what's really bothering you, and explore ways of eliminating the problem.

RECREATION

As we've mentioned in earlier chapters, it's vital to continue involving yourself in the activities you've always enjoyed. Why? Depending on their nature, of course, these activities may help keep you limber and active. Just as important, they will provide a welcome diversion from any worries, prevent boredom and depression, and very likely put you in contact with other people.

Fortunately, most people with prostate cancer are able to participate in their normal recreational activities, including boating, swimming, bowling, golf, tennis, dancing—the list goes on and on. What you do or don't do will depend solely on your own condition—and, of course, on the recommendations of your doctor. If your doctor has given you the green light, and you try an activity without experiencing excessive fatigue, pain, shortness of breath, or other problems, you can feel confident that this activity is okay. On some days, of course, this same sport or pastime may prove to be too much for you. Again, as long as your doctor has given his or her approval, you should let your body be your guide.

ACTIVITIES OF DAILY LIVING

Among the things you do each day are numerous routine tasks—the activities of daily living (ADL). Of course, any restrictions you're experiencing because of prostate cancer may now be limiting these activities. If so, you're probably experiencing a lot of frustration. Why? Because prior to your diagnosis, you most likely took the accomplishment of these simple tasks for granted. And the way you're feeling now, you may be too depressed, upset, or tired to look for a creative solution to these day-to-day problems. (Remember: Not all people with prostate cancer experience these problems. But if you do, it makes sense to see how you can deal with them.)

What should you do? Well, you may not want to ask for help. You may feel that it takes away from your dignity. So you're stuck, right? Absolutely not! In a very short period of time, you can reorganize your lifestyle, your house, and your ADL in a way that will lessen your difficulties and salvage a lot of your dignity. How? Read on!

Simplify Your Tasks

When learning to cope with ADL, keep in mind that your goal is to make daily living as easy as possible in order to conserve energy. You'll want to reduce or eliminate those activities that aren't necessary, and to simplify those that are! (For more about prioritizing tasks, see page 152.) This will allow you to avoid unnecessary fatigue, giving you the energy you require for the things you need—or want—to do.

In many cases, various professionals—physicians or physical therapists, for example—will be able to help you solve any problems you have performing ordinary tasks. But it can be very satisfying to develop your own solutions to these problems.

How can you start? Well, begin by evaluating everything you do on a day-to-day basis. Then see how you can make every single thing you do easier. Is this taking the lazy way out? Of course not. You're simply recognizing that every bit of energy you save in the performance of one activity will give you more energy with which to do something else.

Any specific suggestions? There are lots of things you can do to help yourself with daily living. For instance, you may want to reorganize your home and your habits so that movement becomes easier, and frequently used items are within easy reach. Or you might lubricate drawers so that they open and close more easily. You can wear clothing that is easier to get on and off—Velcro-fastened clothing and sweat suits, for instance. There are also a number of different gadgets that may make life easier for you. For example, you can purchase special devices that will enable you to reach items high on shelves or down on the floor without stretching or bending.

Plan and Organize Your Activities

In addition to eliminating unnecessary activities and making the remaining tasks easier to accomplish, you'll want to learn how to use planning and pacing to conserve energy. Try charting your activities, including both your required tasks and your optional social and leisure activities. This may help you to better organize your time. Certainly, the more advanced the planning the better—especially when big projects are involved—as this will give you time to figure out exactly how you're going to perform a given task, what equipment you'll need, and how the task might be broken up, if necessary, to allow for rest periods. Your local library and bookstores probably contain some excellent books on time management. Many of the tips in these books make such good sense that you'll wonder why you didn't think of them yourself! And every bit of time you save will be a big plus.

A FINAL EXERTION

By now, you've learned a lot about coping with prostate cancer, and you know that staying active is as important as any other coping strategy. You want to feel productive and enjoy life. You don't want to let prostate cancer confine you to your bed or chair. Certainly you should modify any activities that are causing you discomfort, and you should do only what you physically can do, but *do*. . . .

Chapter 24

FINANCIAL PROBLEMS

Having prostate cancer can be a pain in the pocketbook! Why? First, the bills for treatments, laboratory tests, doctor's visits, hospitalization, and other medical services add up. Lost earnings, too, may add to costs—if, for instance, you find that you can work only part-time, or that you must give up work altogether. And if additional help becomes necessary at home, that will also cause expenses to mount. Certainly, the cost for each person—as well as the sources of the costs—varies considerably. But it may not take long for financial security to turn into financial troubles.

Can anything be done to reduce costs or to help pay the ever-mounting bills? Absolutely! Just by taking care of yourself and following your treatment as diligently as possible, you will help to control costs. What else can you do? Let's take a look at the many ways in which you can prevent or ease financial problems as you cope with prostate cancer.

TALK TO OTHERS

If mounting medical costs threaten to engulf you, perhaps the first thing you should do is to speak to other people. Through a support group, for instance, you may be able to meet people in similar situations. Find out what they have done to control and meet the costs of their own care. Even though you may initially be embarrassed to bring up this subject, the common bond that exists among people with medically induced financial problems should quickly put you at ease. You'll be glad you brought it up!

For more ideas, you might contact your physician, hospital administrators, and other health professionals; social workers (see page 210 for more information on federal assistance); and various organizations, such as the American Cancer Society and Cancer Care. Through these contacts, you'll be able to find out which benefits you may be qualified for, and how you can apply for them.

Because financial concerns are such an important part of dealing with cancer, you may wish to include a financial adviser as part of the team of professionals with whom you're working. Your accountant or your insurance agent may be able to help you plan for the future and use your resources as wisely as possible. You might also wish to contact a certified financial planner or chartered financial consultant—listed in the Yellow Pages under "Financial Planning Consultants"—for guidance. Besides advising you about insurance and investments, these experts can tell you about reverse mortgages and other means by which you can borrow money against your assets.

LOWER MEDICATION COSTS

If your treatment includes medication, the use of generic drugs may save you money. Generic medication is sold by its chemical name rather than the more common brand name, and is usually less expensive than the brand-name product. Ask your physician if it would be acceptable to take the generic versions of any drugs you're currently using. If so, your doctor will let your pharmacist know that he or she has okayed the substitution. (Remember, though, that not all generics work as well as their brand-name counterparts!)

ATTEND A CLINIC

If medical costs are overwhelming you, consider attending a clinic. Because clinics usually operate on a sliding-fee schedule, you may be able to get quality medical care at a reduced cost. In some cases, you may even be able to continue seeing the physician who's treating you now, as many physicians donate their time to clinics.

How can you locate a good clinic in your area? Your local hospital or your present physician should be able to guide you to a local clinic that has the resources you need.

INSURANCE CAN BE AN ASSURANCE

Fortunately, many people have some or most of their medical costs defrayed by insurance. What does medical insurance cover? Coverage is usually available for *acute* aspects of the disease—those times when you're actively involved in treatment. In the past, insurance companies were sometimes slow to cover some of the seemingly less significant needs of individuals living with cancer, such as home health care, long-term care, prosthetic devices, and reconstructive surgery. However, because of increased pressures from advocacy organizations, as well as the fact that many more people with cancer are now living longer, more of the costs involved in prostate cancer care are now at least partially covered by insurance.

Most insurance policies have a deductible—an amount of money that you must pay before the insurance coverage begins. In addition, a small percentage of all costs may have to be paid by you, with the insurance company picking up the rest of the tab.

How Can You Get the Most From Your Insurance Policy?

If you have a health-insurance policy, contact your agent as soon as possible, and find out as much as you can about your policy. (The policy itself will provide this information, too, of course.) Ask your agent the amount of your deductible; how many hospital days are covered, and how much is paid per day; how much coverage you have for surgery and anesthesia; whether or not second opinions are covered; and what your maximum lifetime coverage is. Also make sure that you know all of the procedures necessary to file a claim.

How can you help insure that the process of claim filing and reimbursement runs smoothly? If you are responsible for the payment of your insurance premiums, make sure you pay them on time. Don't take the chance of letting your insurance policy lapse. Also be sure to keep track of paperwork. Every time you send in a claim, keep copies of the claim form—and of any attached doctors' bills—for your own files. These may prove invaluable if a problem arises in the processing of your claim. If, in fact, you do not receive a reimbursement on a claim, follow up by phone or letter, and request an explanation of the denial. If no satisfactory response is received, contact the insurance commissioner of your state, requesting an investigation.

Also keep records of the amount your insurance company pays on each claim, as well as the amount *you* pay on each claim. Your own payments may prove to be deductible on your next income tax return. (Your accountant should be able to give you more information on this.)

What If Your Insurance Is Inadequate?

What happens if your insurance coverage is exhausted, or if your insurance is simply not good enough? Well, you may be able to increase the ceiling for your coverage. Additional insurance may also be available for "catastrophic" medical expenses. Be aware, though, that people with cancer often have difficulty obtaining additional health or life insurance. Don't give up, though! It's important to fight any insurance discrimination you're faced with—discrimination that can take the form of cancelled current coverage, reduced benefits, increased premiums, or loss of insurance due to loss of employment.

What If You Have No Health Insurance?

If you are not presently covered by health insurance, you'll want to immediately contact all your resources—your accountant, your lawyer, your financial adviser, and organizations such as the American Cancer Society, for instance—to learn about available options. The more individuals you contact, the more likely it is that you'll find the information you need. Of course, if you are unable to get any insurance coverage and you are also unable to cover your medical costs yourself, you will probably be able to obtain assistance from medicaid. (See page 211 for information.)

GOVERNMENT PROGRAMS MAY HELP

Government insurance programs are an important source of financial support for many people. The type of financial aid program available to you will depend on the type of cancer you have, the type of treatment that you will undergo, your age and financial status, and the eligibility requirements in your area. Let's take a look at the three programs that may prove helpful.

Medicare

Medicare, a federal health insurance program for senior citizens, provides coverage for Americans age sixty-five and over. The degree of coverage provided by medicare varies widely, so it's vital for you to determine exactly what health services medicare will cover in your case.

Medicare is divided into two parts. Part A—which provides coverage for anyone who has reached age sixty-five and is eligible for Social Security benefits—covers hospitalization costs as well as inpatient services in a skilled nursing facility, home health services, and hospice care. No premiums are required for Part A insurance. Part B covers doctor's charges, outpatient hospital services, and specified medical items and services not covered under Part A. Part B insurance, unlike Part A, is voluntary, requiring you to pay a monthly premium. In addition, Part B requires an annual deductible and a 20-percent copayment on your part.

Enrollment in medicare is automatic upon your application for monthly Social Security benefits at age sixty-five. If you decide to continue working past the age of sixty-five, you must apply separately for medicare. Remember, though, that while medicare does provide coverage for large costs, it will not cover everything. Especially in the case of a major illness, supplementary medical coverage is vital.

Medicaid

Medicaid offers benefits to individuals who are unable to pay for health care. This public assistance program is administered on the state or local level. Who qualifies for medicaid? Virtually any low-income individual who demonstrates need can receive these public welfare benefits. If you have any questions about qualifications, or about the benefits themselves, check with your local welfare office for further information.

Social Security Disability Insurance

Disability benefits were added to the Social Security Act in 1956. An individual is considered to be under a disability if he is unable to do *any substantial gainful work* because of a physical or mental impairment; and if the physical or mental condition is expected to last, or has lasted, for at least twelve months, or is expected to result in death. Your eligibility for this coverage will also depend on the stage and site of your cancer. If you are eligible for these benefits, you will receive a fixed monthly benefit, calculated the same way—and equaling the same amount—as your retirement benefits. Your local Social Security office should be able to tell you if you're eligible for disability insurance.

A FINAL $UMMATION

Yes, financial concerns can be a big worry; but despite high costs, most people are able to find ways to pay for appropriate treatment. Certainly, the earlier you start planning, and the more qualified professionals you consult, the greater the likelihood that medical costs will not become a major problem for you. Then you'll be able to concentrate on your most important goal: living successfully with prostate cancer.

Chapter 25

MAKING CHOICES

Most of this book focuses on ways in which you can successfully cope with prostate cancer. The goal, of course, is to do everything you can to live a long, happy, productive life.

Unfortunately, in some cases the disease may be so advanced that you cannot look forward to a long, productive life. You may now be in a position in which you have to face the possibility of premature death. This shouldn't mean, though, that you have to live out the rest of your life in fear. Many people have learned to face the reality of dying, and have coped so well that they've been able to fully enjoy the time left to them.

It can take time to get to the point at which you can accept the possibility of your own death. This adjustment can be a very slow process, and often is emotionally painful, but the results are well worth the effort. Remember that death is certain for everyone. It is only the way in which the remaining days are lived out that varies from person to person. This is where you can reap the greatest benefits.

THE FIVE STAGES OF GRIEVING

Some people know that they are dying well before any professional confirms the fact. Other people do not acknowledge that they are dying until their condition significantly deteriorates or their ability to function significantly changes.

Adjusting to the prospect of death is usually an up-and-down process. There may be times when there is calm acceptance. There may be other times when there are angry "Why me?" reactions. Dr. Elizabeth Kubler-Ross, a psychiatrist who specialized in the psychology of death and dying, developed the concept of the five stages of grieving: denial, anger, bargaining, depression, and acceptance. Family members and close friends may also go through these stages before they are able to more comfortably accept a loved one's condition. In fact, the concept of the five stages is now widely applied to the responses of people who are experiencing any difficult medical problem or other type of tragedy.

Not everyone goes through all five stages of grief. Some people may skip one or more of them, while others may experience the stages in a different order. And some people may spend a lot more time in one stage than in another. It is often comforting to know that reactions such as denial, anger, and depression are normal, and can help you to gradually face the reality of dying.

CHOOSING A COMFORTING ENVIRONMENT

When premature death is likely, a transition must take place from being a person who is fighting for life to being a person who is searching for peace. At this time, the goal is to make the rest of your life—whether it be weeks, months, or years—comfortable. Aggressive medical procedures, which no longer serve any purpose, now are usually discontinued so that the quality of life can be emphasized. This period is much easier when family, friends, and professionals—and you, too—are in agreement as to the new goal. It is far more difficult when there is resistance on the part of any person, whether it is you, a family member, or even a professional.

As part of your efforts to reach your new goal, you will choose the *place* in which you wish to spend your remaining time. Let's look at the two most common options—the hospice and your home.

Hospice Care

A hospice is set up as a warm, comforting place to stay—a place that provides specialized care for individuals whose lives have been shortened by disease. The hospice concept is a comparatively recent one, not having become popular in the United States until the 1970s. Now, many people value the opportunity to spend the autumn of their lives in a hospice facility.

A hospice is one of the best places to obtain palliative treatments—treatments that can make you more comfortable by relieving the pain or other symptoms caused by prostate cancer. For instance, one of the most positive aspects of hospice treatment is the greater availability of painkillers, one form of palliative treatment. Why is pain medication so available in a hospice? Because addiction is no longer a concern. As a result, you are likely to feel more comfortable and be better able to tie up loose ends. Be aware that palliative techniques are not designed to either cure cancer or to suppress its symptoms, as this may no longer be possible.

Hospices may be located within hospitals, or may be separate facilities.

They are designed to provide both treatment for symptoms and psychological counseling—for you and for members of your family. Invariably, the hospice staff is warm, compassionate, and well trained to help residents complete their lives as peacefully and comfortably as possible.

There are many hospice organizations available in local communities. However, if your community does not have such facilities, you can write to the National Hospice Organization at 765 Prospect Street, New Haven, Connecticut 06511, to obtain further information. You can also check with your local chapter of the American Cancer Society.

The costs of hospice care are usually covered by medicare or private insurance carriers. Check with medicare, your nearest Social Security office, or your insurance agent to find out what kind of coverage you have.

Home Care

Despite all of the apparent comforts and benefits of hospice care, many people prefer to spend their remaining days at home. Certainly, familiar surroundings and the care of loved ones can be warm and reassuring.

If you choose to remain at home, make sure that your family is well aware of your wishes, and try to make as many plans as possible while you are able to do so. Social workers and discharge planners at the hospital in which you've been receiving treatment should be able to guide you in making appropriate arrangements, including the rental or purchase of hospital beds or other necessary equipment.

Many of the costs of home care may be covered by private insurance or medicare. Check with the appropriate representatives to find out if nursing, equipment rental, and other costs will be covered in your case.

Emotional Matters

Whether you choose hospice or home care, you should be aware of the emotional turmoil your arrangements may create within your family. To ease any problems, make sure that all family members are included in the decision-making process. These family discussions may pave the way to a more comfortable decision, and may alleviate any possible guilt that could arise on your part as a result of your family's participation in your care. Also, a family that discusses the situation thoroughly and compassionately will be best prepared to deal with any problems that arise over time.

When making your decision, you might want to check with organizations such as the American Cancer Society to obtain the names of people who have used either type of arrangement for their loved ones. In this way, you will be able to make a better-informed decision regarding your own care.

PREPARING FOR THE INEVITABLE

Regardless of the success of your treatment for prostate cancer, death is inevitable for all of us. Yes, you hope that it is something that will happen years and years from now, but your peace of mind may be greatly enhanced if you know that your affairs are in order, and that your family has been provided for in the manner you desire.

In preparing for the inevitable, you'll want to consider five important elements: preparing a valid and up-to-date will; preparing a trust; preparing a letter of instructions that will accompany the will; completing a durable power of attorney document; and preparing a living will. Let's look at each of these components in turn.

The Will

A will guarantees that your property will be distributed according to your wishes; that your estate will be transferred to your heirs with a minimum of delay; and that any young children or other dependents requiring special provisions will be taken care of in the manner you have specified. A will also enables you to designate a legal guardian, who will have the responsibility of caring for or controlling the property of any minor you now care for; a trustee, who will look after the minor's financial interests; and an executor, who will carry out the instructions detailed in your will. Be aware that the same person may fill all three of these roles, or you may choose three different people.

Although it is possible to make out a will on your own, it is certainly not advisable to do so. Only an attorney can guarantee a legally valid will. If you don't already have a lawyer, consider looking for one that specializes in this area of the law.

The Trust

The trust, an important tool of estate planning, is usually set up in the will. A trust is similar to a life insurance policy in that the property held in trust is ultimately distributed to beneficiaries under the terms of the trust agreement. Property received by beneficiaries as the result of the trust will avoid probate, a lengthy and expensive process used to establish the validity of a will and supervise the distribution of assets.

The Supplementary Letter of Instructions

The process of settling an estate begins with the locating of the will and the determining of assets left by the deceased. A supplementary letter of instructions assists the person who will administer the will.

The letter of instructions should state the location of the will, including the names of the lawyer and executor; the names of the people to be notified; the location of vital documents such as certificates of birth and marriage; the location of all assets, including safe deposit boxes and stock and bond certificates; the names of all professional advisers; all employment or business information; and funeral and burial instructions, including wishes regarding disposition of the body and type of service desired. Be sure to include the addresses and telephone numbers of all people mentioned in the letter, so that they can be easily contacted.

The original letter of instructions should be kept with the will, and copies should be given to your spouse and to the will's executor.

Durable Power of Attorney

A durable power of attorney is a document in which you appoint an individual to act as your agent with authority to perform certain specified acts on your behalf in the event that you become disabled or incompetent. Note that this is different from a simple power of attorney, which would terminate immediately upon your incompetency or other disability. Without a durable power of attorney, your physician or hospital would have to search for a family member and ask the court to approve that person's right to act in your behalf.

It may reassure you to know that power of attorney can be revoked by you as long as you remain competent to act. Upon death, the power is automatically revoked. Once this document is complete, give copies to family members, your lawyer, and the executor of your will.

The Living Will

A living will is a document, signed by you, stating that you do not want your life artificially prolonged when it is apparent that death is inevitable. This document must be notarized and signed by witnesses.

When your living will is complete, give copies to your physician and to family members to make sure that your wishes will be followed. It may be beneficial to include the names of these individuals in the living will.

AND SO . . .

Don't give up on the time you have left. Make the most of it. Do what you can to make yourself comfortable and to live life as fully as possible. Make the decisions that seem right to you. And do what you can to give yourself greater peace of mind. Everything we talk about in this book, including the information presented in this chapter, focuses on the importance of improving the quality of your life. It is an achievable goal.

PART V

INTERACTING WITH OTHER PEOPLE

Chapter 26

COPING WITH OTHERS—
AN INTRODUCTION

You do not live your life alone—unless you're reading this book on a deserted island in the Pacific. You interact with many people every day. So you'll certainly want to be able to deal with any difficulties you are having in your interpersonal relationships. For example, you might be worried about what others are going to think now that you've been diagnosed with prostate cancer. How are they going to react? Are they going to ask questions? What kinds of answers will they listen to, and what kinds will turn them away?

Obviously, different kinds of problems exist in different kinds of relationships. But before we begin discussing all the different people who may be part of your life, here are a few general guidelines that you may find helpful.

DO UNTO OTHERS . . .

When you interact with others, try not to get too wrapped up in your own feelings. If you disregard the feelings of those around you, you'll also prevent them from getting close to you. So make a conscious effort to be considerate of others, just as you'd like them to be considerate of you.

What does this mean? Just this: *You're not the only one who has to cope with prostate cancer.* The important people in your life may also be having a hard time, simply because you mean a lot to them. Remember that. You might not realize that your problems affect those around you. You might think, "Why would they be upset? It's happening to me!" But if you give this some thought, you'll see that you're not being reasonable or fair.

Take your family, for example. A problem for you is also a problem for them. Of course, it may affect you in a different way. It's certainly true that you're the one who's experiencing the restrictions and the physical changes, as well as the apprehensions and anxieties. But your family doesn't like to see you suffer. You'll be better able to cope with these important people if you bear in mind that they are experiencing almost as much emotional turmoil as you are. In fact, this may explain why family members and friends might be unable to provide all of the support you want as quickly as you want it. Like you, they are probably going through a tough period of adjustment!

Then again, rather than being unaware of the emotions of others, you may feel guilty about the added burden you are placing on your family. This can be a hard feeling to cope with. Keep in mind, though, that you may be projecting this difficulty on to other people—and possibly adding to their problems in the process. Chances are, they don't feel as burdened as you may fear. They may feel temporarily helpless or overwhelmed, but still be eager to help.

CHANGE YOURSELF, NOT OTHERS

Do you feel that if you try hard enough, you'll be able to change the attitudes, feelings, or behaviors of others? Unfortunately, it doesn't work that way. Whether the people in your life accept your prostate cancer or deny that you have any problem at all, you won't be able to change them unless they want to change. So it makes sense to use your energy to change the one person over whom you *do* have control—yourself. Spend more time working on yourself, and less time worrying about others. In fact, once others see the changes in you, they may even alter their own attitudes. So help yourself. Be your own best friend.

LOOK THROUGH THE EYES OF OTHERS

If you have an argument with someone, you may believe that you're right and the other person is wrong. If this continues, nothing will be resolved, and the other person's behavior may drive you crazy because it seems so unreasonable.

Take a moment, and look at the situation through the eyes of the other person. What does he or she see? What might the other point of view be? Once you've looked through the eyes of the other person, you'll be better able to explain how you feel in a way that he or she will understand. And then you'll be able to find a solution to almost any problem that might exist.

LEARN TO SAY "NO"

Perhaps you've been feeling rotten, but others seem to want you to do more and more. In the past, you may have had trouble saying "no"—because you felt guilty, perhaps, or because you wanted to avoid disappointing the other person. Now, though, things are a little different, and you really must curtail your generosity for the sake of your own well-being. Yes, this may mean your giving the appearance of being selfish. But as long as you don't abuse it, this selfishness can be positive for you. Do for yourself; think of yourself. You're Number One, and that's the way it must be. Only if you take care of yourself will you be able to deal with others. The reverse does not necessarily hold true. If you always take care of others first, this may actually make you *less* able to care for yourself.

DEVELOP A STRONG SUPPORT SYSTEM

You'll find it far easier to deal with prostate cancer if you can rely on those closest to you, such as your spouse, other family members, and close friends. This social network can give you added strength during this difficult time.

However, you should anticipate that when you first let those close to you know what's going on, you may sense a distancing. As we've already discussed, this will not occur because others don't want to help you. They probably do. However, it may be difficult for them to deal with your condition, especially right after the diagnosis. They may be fearful of the possibility of your dying, or they may feel helpless, or even feel angry because your situation has created additional problems for them. Try to anticipate this, and to recognize that they are simply coming to grips with a problem—a problem that you're working to adjust to, also. Eventually, they should be better able to help you.

If you find that you don't have the kind of social network that you would like to have, it may be helpful to get involved in a support group. There, you will meet people who can provide the caring and understanding that you need to cope with prostate cancer. (For information on support groups, see Chapter 9.)

OPEN THE LINES OF COMMUNICATION

We've just discussed how the support and understanding of others can help you deal better with your new problems. But right now, you may find it difficult to even *talk* to others. So how can you possibly ask for their support? Well, your first job is to get the lines of communication open. And how can you do that? The best way to get the conversation rolling is to be open and honest about the way you feel. If you say anything that upsets or hurts somebody else, you'll deal with it then. But first, get your feelings out on the table.

Perhaps you're waiting for others to approach you and offer their support. But since you're the one with cancer, you may have to be the first person to talk about it. Other people may be reluctant to even mention the word in front of you. If you bring it up and talk about it matter-of-factly, you may ease the way to very effective communication.

What if you're too fearful to share your feelings? Certainly, fear can make communication difficult, if not impossible. For instance, if you're fearful that what you have to say may embarrass the other person, you may hesitate to say it. Or perhaps it's their fear that's stopping you. Fortunately, there's an excellent solution to this problem. Simply reach out and physically touch the other person. By holding hands or sharing hugs, you can quickly bring about a type of sharing that doesn't require words. And in the process, you'll reestablish the lines of communication.

BRING ON THE WORLD

Now that we've introduced some general ideas, let's see how prostate cancer can affect the different relationships that may be part of your life. Of course, not every chapter in this section will apply to you. You may choose to read only those that are appropriate, or you may decide to read all the chapters. However you choose to approach this material, you'll soon realize that problems exist in all relationships, but that these problems—like most problems—can be coped with successfully.

Chapter 27

YOUR FAMILY

Blood is thicker than water! Your family can be a critical factor in your successful adjustment to prostate cancer. Why? You're probably with your family more than you're with anyone else. If you get along well with members of your family, you have a ready source of emotional and practical support.

The impact of your prostate cancer on your family is sure to be profound. It seems that family members who are able to talk, share, cry, and hold on to each other during rough times have an easier time dealing with the problems posed by cancer. On the other hand, when family members experience the impact but are unable to talk to one another about it, the adjustment is much more difficult. Which of these families sounds like yours? If your family is like most, it falls somewhere in between these two extremes.

Any communication problems that exist within a family are usually magnified by cancer. The fact that different people adjust at different speeds—and may have varying degrees of difficulty in dealing with change—can also exacerbate family problems.

If you find it difficult to talk to loved ones about your cancer, its prognosis, or its treatment, don't give up. To maintain family unity—and to make sure you get the support that you need—it's important that your concerns be brought into the open. This doesn't mean that all conversations are going to be pleasant. However, they should enable each person to share his or her feelings with the other members of the family.

Of course, different types of problems may pop up with different family members. So let's discuss how you can better deal with your wife, your children, and your parents.

LIVING WITH YOUR WIFE

Prostate cancer can certainly have an effect on your marriage. But this doesn't mean that your problems can't be resolved. There are very few problems that can't be worked out through better communication, understanding, and, if necessary, counseling. Let's discuss some of the ways in which a marriage can show the impact of prostate cancer, as well as various ways in which this impact can be lessened.

Changes in Your Social Life

Have the restrictions caused by prostate cancer forced you to cut back on some of the social activities you used to enjoy with your wife? You might not be able to do as much now as you used to. This can be hard to take, especially if you and your spouse had active social lives before the onset of your condition. Because your wife does not have prostate cancer, she may feel angry, frustrated, or helpless. You, on the other hand, may feel that you're a burden on your wife. Or you may be angered by her seeming inability to accept these new restrictions.

Probably, once your condition stabilizes, you'll be able to resume many of your usual activities. Until then, try to engage in activities that require minimal physical energy with people who are flexible enough to handle last-minute changes. Sometimes, just watching a video with a few friends can be a pleasant experience.

If, however, your social life is still on hold even after your condition has stabilized, you'll have to ask yourself if this is due to fear, depression, or other emotional problems. If so, refer to the appropriate chapters earlier in the book.

Changes in Family Responsibilities

Prostate cancer may create the need for temporary or permanent changes in each family member's responsibilities as your spouse and children take over some of the functions that you performed in the past. This can surely be another potential source of friction between you and your wife, especially if she receives a heavy share of the load.

Lorraine, a forty-six-year-old mother of three, was told by her husband, fifty-two-year-old Wayne, that she would have to take over many of her husband's responsibilities—such as mowing the lawn, caring for the garden, paying the bills, and balancing the checkbook—because he no longer had the necessary energy (or interest). Because of this, their two teen-age children would have to help out with the grocery shopping and cooking. Despite the fact that Wayne's family loved him and was concerned about his health, his wife and children were understandably upset. His wife was especially upset, since she knew little about the new tasks she was expected to accomplish.

How can you make changes as smoothly as possible, without causing your wife unnecessary distress? First, make the changes gradually. Try to avoid overwhelming your wife—or other members of your family, for that matter. And be realistic in your expectations, keeping in mind that it may take time for your wife to comfortably incorporate her new responsibilities into her routine.

How else can you help your spouse adjust to greater burdens? Make sure that free time is still available for the pleasures of life. It's only when new responsibilities seem to be all-consuming that serious problems may occur. Be sure to look at any changes through the eyes of your wife. Consider how you'd feel if the situation were reversed. Think how upsetting it would be if you no longer had time for the things you enjoyed because of added responsibilities and pressures. Discuss the needed changes reasonably, and be gentle. Just as important, as these changes occur, be gentle with yourself. When you see other members of your family taking over certain responsibilities, you may feel more and more hopeless and worthless. Look at this situation as being temporary.

If Your Wife Denies Your Condition

What can you do if your wife simply won't accept the fact that you have prostate cancer? You can, of course, try to "educate" your spouse, but try not to go overboard. If you're constantly badgering your wife and reminding her of the things that must change because of your condition, you may only cause her to further deny the problem. Keep in mind that your wife will not accept your condition until she is ready to do so. In the meantime, concentrate on improving your own thoughts and feelings. Others' feelings may change, but they will do so slowly, and probably not at your urgings.

Financial Problems

Prostate cancer can present added money problems, especially if your wife previously had little to do with family finances, and now must share or take charge of financial responsibilities. But even if your wife has always taken part in the family's money matters, medical bills—and possibly a newly reduced income—can make things tough. Both you and your spouse may worry whether all obligations can be met, and whether they will continue to be met over time. Of course, money concerns are a source of friction in many marriages. Here, though, the problem is compounded.

What can you do? Sit down with your wife and talk over your financial problems. Try to be realistic and to reach practical solutions. Admit that new problems may arise, but emphasize the fact that they frequently have a way of working themselves out. If not, you will deal with them as they come. Be patient, be communicative, and above all, be positive.

Has Your Sex Life Been Affected?

As you've learned in previous chapters—and as you may know from your own experience—prostate cancer can affect sexual relations. If this is a problem for you and your wife, or if you'd just like to learn more about the possible impact that prostate cancer can have on sex, see Chapter 31. In that chapter, you'll learn how sexual problems can be worked out so that sex can remain an important and pleasurable part of your life.

In Sickness and in Health? Sorry!

Unfortunately, some marriages have ended because of chronic medical problems. Cancer-related restrictions, fears, symptoms, and side effects certainly have the potential to drive a wedge into what may have previously been a good relationship, replacing feelings of closeness and intimacy with coldness and distance. This can wash the "magic" right out of a marriage.

What should you do if your wife is frightened and "wants out"? First, be aware that any problems in the marriage may not be entirely your wife's fault. For instance, you may feel too apprehensive to enjoy your relationship, and your and your wife's combined problems may be creating a horrible package of anxiety, depression, and panic. What should you do after you try to view the problem objectively? Get help. This package isn't one you can—or should—handle alone, and if communication has become a problem in your house, you may not be able to talk to your wife. The aid of a professional or an objective outsider may help to resolve some of the problems that you and your wife have been unable to solve yourselves. If possible, include your mate in your counseling sessions. But once again, don't force the issue. If your wife doesn't seem open to outside help, get some counseling for yourself. Regardless of the results of your efforts to save your marriage, any support you can muster will only improve your emotional well-being.

A Marital (Con)Summation

Every marriage has its ups and downs, with problems that have to be worked out. Of course, prostate cancer does make relationships more vulnerable to crises and arguments. In fact, at this point, it may seem very difficult, or even impossible, to deal with your wife. But by giving added attention to your wife's feelings and needs, you will find that many—if not all—of these problems can be worked out over time. And I think you'll agree that your relationship is worth the added effort. Once problem spots have been smoothed out and necessary adjustments have been eased, your wife may become your greatest ally in dealing with your condition.

LIVING WITH YOUR CHILDREN

Children—regardless of how old they are!—may be particularly vulnerable to the stresses and fears that occur when a family member has cancer. Certainly, at this time, you may not be able to help them as much as you used to, or to spend as much time with them as you'd like. But you can surely use the time you do spend with them as productively as possible, and you can also do a great deal to help your children more easily handle any fears or changes that may be bothering them. How? Let's see how you can cope with your children, and how you can help them to better cope with your condition.

Encourage Questions

When you talk to your children, make sure that you take time to answer any questions they may have. Discussions, if handled properly, will not only be helpful for your children, but can also provide both you and your kids with a special feeling of closeness.

But what if your kids don't ask questions? Remember that if your children really don't want to, they won't, no matter how much encouragement you give them. But you should let them know that they can ask you anything they want, as fears can get more and more destructive if kept inside. Once your kids know that they have the option of talking to you freely, they can decide what, if anything, they wish to discuss.

How should you answer your children's questions? This depends on the ages of your kids, as well as on how detailed an answer they're looking for. The best advice is to provide direct answers to each question. Don't go into detail unless your children ask for more information. Try to determine exactly what your kids want to know. This may be tricky, as even your children may not know what answers they're looking for. So just start talking, and provide them with more information as they ask for it.

Should you explain prostate cancer to your children? Again, this depends partly on the ages of your kids. With very young children, you might just say, "I don't feel well, so I can't play catch. I'd like to, but I just can't." Unless your condition is advanced, you may decide not to say much of anything. With older children, of course, explanations can be more detailed.

Certainly, whenever you're speaking to your children about illness—especially if your kids are young—you should be careful not to frighten them. Remember that children have great imaginations, and often blow things out of proportion. You do want your kids to continue talking to you about your condition. If you show that you accept prostate cancer—as much as you can—and that you welcome questions about it, this will greatly benefit your relationship with your kids.

Of course, there's one question your children might ask that will be particularly hard to answer. Whenever children know that a parent has a serious medical problem, they may worry, and may ask if the parent is going to die. You'll have to handle this very carefully. Children become petrified thinking about the death of a parent. So unless your condition has already become advanced, reassure them as best you can that you're not going to die. These may seem like empty words, but, at this time, that's what your kids need to hear. You'll deal with any changes in this "prognosis" if and when it becomes necessary to do so.

If you have difficulty discussing your illness with your children, it might be a good idea to speak to a professional—your doctor or your children's doctor, for example—and have him or her take control of the discussion.

Focus on Quality, Not Quantity

Prostate cancer can be restrictive. Fatigue, pain, and uncomfortable side effects—not to mention treatment schedules and surgery—may prevent you from doing a lot of what you'd like to do. Yet, especially now, you may want to spend as much time as possible with your children. How can you solve this dilemma? Honestly explain to your children that you're not able to do as much as you'd like to. Then come to an agreement with them about some enjoyable activity you can share with them when you're feeling better. This arrangement will show your children that you're aware of their unhappiness, and that you do want to spend more time with them.

Also try to be less concerned with *quantity time*—the number of minutes and hours you spend with your kids—and more concerned with *quality time*—special time during which you share feelings and pleasurable activities. If your time together is well spent, with plenty of talking and laughing, it will make up for any missed time. And as you share your thoughts with your children, you'll be helping them to better handle your medical condition.

Adolescents

During adolescence, children begin to assert their independence. Look out, world! The future generation is coming! Adolescents want to start moving away from the family setting and its responsibilities. Even under normal circumstances, this creates problems in many homes. Add a parent with prostate cancer to the picture, and the problem is compounded. Why? Because of your condition, your teen may have to help out more than usual around the house. At the same time, he or she probably wants to do less around the house, and be away more. How can you cope with this predicament? Well, in truth, you may not be able to change your teen much. But perhaps you can learn to cope in a way that, at the very least, keeps you sane! Let's learn more about dealing with teens.

Don't Expect Miracles!

First, realize that dealing with teens is quite different from dealing with younger kids—which you probably already know. As already discussed, teens are absorbed far more in themselves than in their family. Remember that they are going through quite a few difficult adjustments on their own, and seem to have little interest in others—*especially* their parents! Of course, not all teens are alike. Some are less self-centered and more sensitive and compassionate than others. Certainly, you know your child better than anyone. But perhaps you expect your usually insensitive child to rise to the occasion and enthusiastically pitch in with household chores. Be aware that you are probably setting yourself up for disappointment if you expect your child to change significantly.

Of course, this doesn't mean that you shouldn't discuss your condition with your teen. Talk to your child candidly, treating him or her like an adult, as this will probably provide the best chance of a good response. Think about the concerns your adolescent might have regarding the prostate cancer, and try to be reassuring. If your teen feels comfortable talking to you about your condition, encourage discussion. But remember to respect the rights of those adolescents who would rather not talk about your illness. And, again, don't expect miracles, and don't let yourself be devastated if your adolescent shows little interest.

When You Need Your Teen to Pitch In

Because of your condition, your adolescent may now have to shoulder more responsibilities. But will your teen be willing to help out? That's the real question!

Seventeen-year-old Melissa, whose father had been diagnosed with prostate cancer, felt guilty about not helping out more at home, but thought that giving in would be a sign of weakness. (Heaven forbid!) This caused Melissa a lot of anguish—which, of course, she didn't want to discuss with her parents. Because of the guilt she was experiencing, Melissa escaped by spending even more time than usual out of the house—and less time helping out! Melissa's parents sat her down, and together they worked out a compromise. Melissa would not have to spend all her time helping out at home, but she would make herself available when necessary. After reaching an agreement, Melissa and her folks felt closer to one another—and Melissa felt a good deal better about herself.

So, you see, it may pay to take the initiative and offer a reasonable compromise. Just showing that you understand your teen's feelings may help. Perhaps things won't seem so hopeless to your child, after all.

Another tactic, too, may prove helpful. If your adolescent must take on some adult chores, consider that he or she may be ready to enjoy a few adult privileges and pleasures—within reason, of course. Certainly, adolescents are usually more willing to help out if they know that they will be treated and trusted in a more grown-up way.

Remember that you can go only so far in trying to get your adolescent's cooperation. You can't move mountains. Continue to be as constructive as you can, putting as little pressure on your child as possible in order to keep the door open to good relations. As long as you know you've tried, you can hold your head up high.

DEALING WITH YOUR PARENTS

Parents often have difficulty coping with their child's illness—even if their "child" is an adult. Certainly, something as serious as prostate cancer is hard to take. Therefore, if your parents are alive, anticipate that they'll have a rough time. This, of course, will make coping harder for you, too. Why? You don't want your parents to suffer. And you know how your parents feel, because you'd certainly be upset if any child of yours was ill.

If your relationship with your parents is good, then you're among the lucky ones. But what if you normally have difficulty dealing with your parents? Having prostate cancer won't help! But regardless of the type of relationship you've had previously, consider how your parents have treated you since your diagnosis. Have they ignored or minimized your condition? Or have they smothered you? Let's look at these two possible reactions, and see how you can better cope with your parents.

The Ignorers

Since Pat's diagnosis with prostate cancer two years before, his parents had shown less and less concern about his condition. Whenever Pat mentioned that he had pain, his mother just told him to "call the doctor." When Pat was tired, his father told him that "staying in bed won't accomplish anything." If looks could kill . . . ! Other than making these insensitive remarks, Pat's parents had little to say on the subject of his prostate cancer. They certainly never asked questions about his condition. Even worse, when he did try to fill them in, they showed no interest at all.

Parents who ignore or play down your medical condition often do so because they can't deal with your illness. They can't face the fact that their child is sick. (And it doesn't matter how old you are!) Worse, many parents agonize over the possibility that your problem might have something to do with them. While this may not make any sense to you, your parents may be afraid that they did something to contribute to your illness, or that you inherited the condition from them. To avoid these intolerable thoughts, they may try to deny your having prostate cancer, or they may minimize your illness, hoping it will all go away.

Remember what we said in the previous chapter about how it helps to see a situation through someone else's eyes? Don't you think that it holds true in this case? As you look through the eyes of your seemingly indifferent parents, you'll probably realize that this is the only way in which they can cope with the situation right now. Yes, their behavior may change over time, but the change will be gradual, and will not necessarily be in response to your urgings.

The Smotherers

After David was told that he had prostate cancer, his mother began visiting him on the average of four times a week. This would have been nice, except: (1) His mother lived forty-five minutes away by car. (2) His mother had emphysema and needed her rest. (3) David simply didn't want to see her so often. You see, David was sixty-one, hadn't lived at home for forty years, and often disagreed with his mother—especially regarding how much he should do and how much rest he should get. David certainly felt smothered.

Parents who smother believe that if you have any kind of problem, they must take care of you. Having prostate cancer certainly fits this requirement. It doesn't matter what your marital status is, or how old you are, or if you can take of yourself. What matters to them is that they are your parents—they are responsible for your welfare. They'll call frequently, asking how you're doing. They'll want to know what they can do to help. They may come over as often as possible to make sure you're okay. Whether they visit or not, they'll constantly bombard you with questions about your health and activities.

What can you do, short of moving out of town and taking on a new identity? Again, look at yourself—and your condition—through the eyes of your parents. How do you think they feel? They care about you. What do you see? They see a child who needs them! You may not agree with them, but understanding their point of view should help you explain how you feel.

What If Talking Doesn't Help?

If you have talked to your parents and haven't succeeded in modifying their behavior, at least you know you've tried. This, alone, may help you feel better! What else can you do? Right! Concentrate on helping yourself feel better. If your folks are unhappy with you because you seem to be rejecting their well-meaning intentions, so be it. If your folks are unhappy with you because you're making it hard for them to ignore your condition, so be it.

By the way, if you're unhappy with parents who are ignorers, you'd probably love them to smother you for a while. And if you don't like smothering parents, the thought of being left alone is probably very appealing. There's rarely a perfect situation or relationship, and no one gets along with everyone all the time. Instead of complaining about your parents' faults, try to look at the positives in their behavior. This may make you feel better, and will certainly help you avoid going crazy over your parents' actions.

How Much Should You Tell Your Parents?

A common question of people with chronic conditions concerns how much they should tell their parents about their problem. Have you been worrying about this, too? First, think about your parents. How do they usually deal with unpleasant situations? Then ask yourself what, precisely, you want to share with them. Then imagine how they would react to this, and how you would handle their reactions. All these factors will help you decide how much you should tell them.

For instance, you might wish you could share your fears and worries with your parents because of the reassurances it would bring. It certainly would be nice to know that you don't have to face something unpleasant alone. But what if your parents couldn't readily accept your problems even if they wanted to? It might be more detrimental to tell them things that they couldn't handle. So don't impulsively blurt your feelings out. By spending a little time figuring out what's best, you will help yourself feel a lot better. You'll probably improve your relationship with your parents, as well.

Finally, keep in mind that it's sometimes easier to talk to one parent than to the other. Consider telling one parent what's bothering you, and letting that parent tell the other. For example, your mother may be able to get through to your father better than you can. This will make things easier for everybody.

A FAMILIAL CONCLUSION

As you learn to cope with prostate cancer, your biggest allies—a source of emotional support and practical assistance—may be your family. By learning to deal with your family members in the best possible way, you'll not only make things easier for them, but you'll also make them better able to help you cope with prostate cancer.

Chapter 28

FRIENDS
AND COLLEAGUES

Aside from family, other people you deal with on a daily, or nearly daily, basis are friends and colleagues. Are there any ways in which you can better deal with these important people? Of course!

DEALING WITH YOUR FRIENDS

Cancer can certainly teach you who your real friends are. Those people you thought were close to you may prove to be not so close. And those people you liked but didn't think would be there for you may, in a pinch, prove to be your most supportive allies. And you can always try to meet new friends, as well. In fact, prostate cancer may even help this to happen. How? If you join a support group for individuals with cancer, you may meet new and interesting people with whom you have much in common.

Perhaps, before your diagnosis, your relationships with your friends were fairly effortless. Unfortunately, prostate cancer may have changed that. You may be surprised—even hurt—by the seeming aloofness of some friends, while other friends may be too supportive. Then, of course, there are the special problems that may crop up because of your condition—activities cancelled because of fatigue, or the need to ask for help. These are problems that can exact a toll on seemingly strong friendships. How can you handle this? Read on!

Be Prepared for Different Reactions

How have your friends reacted to your prostate cancer? How many even know what prostate cancer is all about? They may have read about it, and, at first, they may have thought they understood prostate cancer.

But because they haven't been directly affected by the disorder, they may not be able to really understand what you are experiencing. Some may want to learn more; some may want to forget what little they already know.

Certainly you should be prepared for a variety of reactions to your condition. Some friends, for instance, may seem uninterested and distant. Why would a friend seem distant at a time when you need special support? Well, some people may not know what to say to you. Their heads may be filled with doubts and questions. What should they ask you? How should they talk to you? Should they even mention your condition? They may not want to run the risk of stirring up unpleasant feelings for you—or for themselves, if they don't know how to respond. Their doubts and fears may cause so much tension that they don't even want to be with you.

Of course, some friends may be very supportive—maybe too supportive! There may be times when friends keep asking you how you are, or offering help when you'd simply like to be left alone.

Certainly, friendships can be hurt or lost because of misunderstandings and uncertainties. Can anything be done to prevent these problems from undermining your friendships, or are you going to be a hermit for the rest of your life? Don't despair. There are things you can do to improve the situation.

Try to establish ground rules with your friends. If you're the kind of person who likes to be asked how you feel and wants friends around you at all times, let your friends know. If you'd rather not be asked about your health, let them know that, too. If your feelings fluctuate—if you sometimes feel talkative about your condition, but at other times prefer not to even think about it—make your friends aware of this. Of course, you should realize that this may be difficult for your friends, who will have no way of knowing how you feel at any given time. So tell them that they should simply say what's on their minds. You'll let them know if and when you're having trouble.

Clear up the question marks. If you tell your friends what your needs and desires are, fewer unknowns will exist. The uneasiness about what to do or say, as well as the fear of saying or doing the wrong thing, will be reduced. Communication will be easier, and you and your friends will feel a great deal closer.

Changing Plans

Don't you love having to change plans with a friend at the last minute because you're so worn out that you can't even move? Probably not. So you can understand how your friends might feel about it. However, good friends, who understand or at least try to understand what you're going through, will probably be able to accept these last-minute cancellations.

Ken hated having to bow out of plans with friends because of the side effects of his prostate cancer treatments. He felt guilty about letting his friends down, and at the same time resented their annoyance over the cancellations, as well as their apparent lack of understanding. Ken decided to sit down with some of his closest friends and work out a solution to the problem. He even asked them for suggestions. Ken's friends thought that he should participate only in nonstrenuous activitiesactivities that he would be most likely to follow through on. The discussion brought about a greater closeness for all involved, as well as greater empathy for Ken's situation.

In your case, you may not always get the understanding you want. But you'll probably find at least one or two friends who will be willing to work on a solution to any problems.

Asking for Help

As you learn to live with prostate cancer, you may have a greater need to call on your friends for help. Are you becoming more selfish? No—although it may seem that way to you. You'd probably like to be able to do these things yourself, but it just may not be possible. The reality is that there are certain things that must be taken care of, and if you can't take care of them yourself, you must ask others to help you. So if you need help, reach out for it. That's better than pushing yourself too much and suffering the consequences.

When planning to ask a friend for help, keep in mind that older friendships tend to be stronger and more resilient. Such friends will probably be more receptive when approached for favors. Newer or more casual friends should probably not be burdened as much. Without giving a friendship a chance to become firmly planted on your hook, you may lose your prize fish—a good, long-lasting friendship. Also base your choice on the type of help you need. Aim for a proper fit. (By the way, no matter how old and dear the friend, when you feel up to it, it would be nice to show your appreciation through an unexpected gift or gesture.)

What should you do if your friends complain or show resentment when you request help? Back off for a while. In addition, try to talk it over with them. Discuss these problems when the conflict can still be resolved; don't let them build up until the friendship is destroyed. If your efforts to mend the friendship fail, remember this: Friends who can't understand your need for help are not very good friends, anyway.

Losing Friends

What if the people you thought were your friends don't call or visit? What if they seems reluctant to make any plans with you, preferring to "wait and see how you feel." When friends seem to drift away, it's certainly sad. But remember that it was not your decision to end the friendship. And you don't want it to be your problem!

Why might this have happened? Maybe your friend felt uncomfortable about being with you. Maybe he was "turned off" by the fact that you have a medical problem. Or perhaps he was unsure of what to say or do. Whatever the reason, you've probably learned a hard, unpleasant lesson: You can't change someone else's feelings.

If a friend, or anyone else, cannot handle your condition, you may feel rejected. This can be devastating—especially if you fear that you won't be able to develop any other meaningful relationships! This is not true. You are the same person you were before your diagnosis. Keep telling yourself this so that you can restore any confidence that may have been shaken by your friend's action. Be reassured that most people who lose friends do make new ones. Anyway, you really don't want a "friend" who is uncomfortable around you. You want a friend who likes you the way you are, prostate cancer and all! And there are plenty of wonderful, understanding people out there. So don't give up!

DEALING WITH YOUR COLLEAGUES

If you work, you're probably spending many hours a week with a number of colleagues. These colleagues are likely to show a variety of reactions to your condition (if they know about it), as well as to any impact your condition may be having on your work. Let's discuss some of the ways in which you may better cope with your colleagues.

Should You Tell Your Colleagues?

Hopefully, if you're comfortable with yourself, others will be, too. Many colleagues will take your condition in stride, and won't even think about it. Might it be helpful to provide your colleagues with some basic information on prostate cancer? It could be, although you should realize that this would not necessarily improve their attitude toward you or your condition. Unfortunately, knowledge doesn't always lead to understanding. However, just knowing that you've tried to help your colleagues understand might make you feel better.

Of course, unless nosy colleagues ask questions, you may decide not to even bother telling your co-workers about your condition. Obviously, there is no requirement that you do so. And your co-workers probably won't see any evidence of prostate cancer—unless they have x-ray vision!

When Colleagues Are Resentful

Tom was a fifty-eight-year-old accountant who had worked in the same office for twenty-two years. Because of prostate cancer, Tom found it necessary to reduce his eight-hour-a-day work schedule to four hours. This plan was endorsed by his physician and employer, but was not accepted graciously by his fellow workers, many of whom would have preferred similar part-time arrangements! This caused bitterness and strain in Tom's working relationships.

If you have to curtail your working hours, or if you find that you must miss work frequently because of prostate cancer, you, like Tom, may encounter some resentment. As discussed above, at this point you may decide to explain your situation to your colleagues, or you may prefer to keep this information to yourself. Either way, accept the fact that some people just won't *want* to understand what's happening to you and why. Remember: You can't change somebody else. If a colleague—or anybody else, for that matter—can't handle or understand what's going on, that's his or her problem. You can try to educate people about prostate cancer, but you shouldn't make their attitude your problem. If you've got an employer with an open mind, you're way ahead of the game. Don't be as concerned about the attitudes of other people. Instead, concentrate on doing what's best for you.

Cooperative Colleague Compromises

Occasionally, you may find yourself unable to complete all of your work. When this happens, try to make some kind of arrangement with a colleague. What type of arrangement might you make? Certainly, it depends on the relationship between you and the other person, as well as on the type and amount of work that needs to be done. You might, for instance, offer to pay your co-worker for completing your assignment. Or you might take over some of his or her responsibilities when you can.

This type of arrangement may seem strange—even uncomfortable—at first, but it can result in even better relationships between you and your colleagues. You have nothing to lose. The worst your co-worker can say is, "No! I won't help."

Whether you need to work or you simply enjoy working, you'll certainly want to minimize any potential occupational problems caused by your condition. And you'll certainly want to maintain good friendships so that you can continue to involve yourself in interesting and emotionally supportive social activities.

Whether dealing with co-workers or with friends, always make sure to take one day at a time. Don't worry about problems that have not yet occurred—and, for that matter, may never occur. If and when your prostate cancer does cause a problem, be precise in identifying exactly what the problem is. Then don't hesitate to employ the best strategies you know to resolve the dilemma, and to restore good relations between you and the people you deal with in your day-to-day life.

Chapter 29

YOUR PHYSICIAN

How do you feel about your physician? (What a question!) Some people see physicians as gods. Others feel that they're rich, indifferent, cold professionals who don't really want to help. Your view of your doctor will help determine how your treatment progresses. You may find that your feelings towards your physician—or towards physicians in general—have changed since your diagnosis. Some people with prostate cancer don't have as much confidence in their physicians, probably because they haven't been cured yet! Others see them as being their "last hope." Let's learn more about the doctor-patient relationship, and see how you can improve your dealings with your own physician.

FINDING THE RIGHT DOCTOR

Many individuals with prostate cancer question which type of doctor they should be working with. The consensus is that a urologist—a physician who specializes in disorders of the urinary and genital tracts—is the most appropriate doctor, since a urologist is most familiar with prostate cancer, its symptoms, and its treatment. However, other specialists—radiation oncologists, for instance—may also be involved, depending on your particular condition.

During your treatment, your primary physician will be the hub of the wheel. Your primary physician will—hopefully—be your advocate in determining which treatments will be best for you, both now and in the future. He or she will also help coordinate the efforts of any other physicians with whom you'll be working. This doctor will help you manage your symptoms, help decrease the risk of complications, give you guidelines for any lifestyle changes that may be beneficial or necessary, and even work with you when medical problems unrelated to cancer occur during your treatment.

What should you look for when choosing your primary physician—or when choosing any physician, for that matter? First, you'll want someone in whom you have confidence medically. The reason for this is clear. But, just as important, you'll want someone with whom you're comfortable personally. You see, research has suggested that the more comfortable you are with your physician, the more likely you'll be to comply with prescribed treatment, and the better you may respond to this treatment. And, of course, you must remember that you'll have to see your physician a good deal more often than would someone who doesn't have a chronic medical problem.

A great many factors will determine your ability to feel comfortable with your physician, including your personality, your doctor's personality, your age, your doctor's age, your doctor's philosophy regarding treatment, and more. Remember that the chemistry between a doctor and each patient is unique. Although a friend or relative may recommend the "perfect" doctor, he or she may not be right for you. You'll have to pick somebody whom *you* feel good about.

When seeing a doctor for the first time, there are a number of questions you may want answered to determine if this physician is right for you. The following queries should get you started in the right direction.

- [ ] Is the doctor an expert in the field of prostate cancer, and has he or she had a good deal of experience treating individuals with this disorder?
- [ ] Is the doctor's office located close enough to your home to enable you to visit the office easily at those times when you're not feeling well?
- [ ] What are the doctor's hours? Are they convenient for you? How long does it take to schedule an appointment?
- [ ] How long will it take the doctor to call you back when you phone him or her with a question? Also, will you always receive a return call from your own doctor, or will you sometimes have to talk to an associate?
- [ ] What are the anticipated fees? What are the doctor's policies regarding insurance?
- [ ] How supportive and cooperative is the doctor's staff? (You may find this question surprising. However, many people change doctors simply because of difficulties encountered with the office staff!)
- [ ] Does the doctor genuinely seem concerned about you as a person?
- [ ] If you have an interest in alternative treatments, what are the doctor's views on the subject? Is he or she dead set against alternative therapies, open-minded on the subject, or very familiar with the available options?

☐ Is the doctor willing and able to answer your questions in language that you find understandable?

Of course, we all want the perfect doctor—the doctor with the best credentials, the most experience, the most impressive reputation, and the warmest bedside manner. (And, of course, the office should be right around the corner!) But accept the fact that you probably won't be able to find a doctor who meets all of your criteria, and try to focus on what's most important to you. You may, for instance, be willing to accept a doctor whose manner is a little cold if his qualifications are excellent and his approach to treatment is in line with your own philosophy. Use your judgment, and make the decision with which you feel most comfortable.

CREATING A GOOD DOCTOR-PATIENT RELATIONSHIP

Once you've chosen your primary physician—and, possibly, other doctors as well—you'll want to make sure that the relationship with your doctor gets off to a good start and continues on track. Fortunately, there are two things you can do to help make—and keep—your relationship pleasant and, most important, beneficial.

Set Communication Ground Rules

It's vital to set ground rules regarding your communication with your doctor. In the past, it was a popularly held belief that patients with cancer wanted to know as little as possible, so doctors tried to minimize the amount of information they shared. Today, this is usually not the case. Many people want to be very actively involved in their treatment, and want all the facts. However much information you want, make sure to clearly communicate your needs to your doctor. Of course, this is a fairly simple matter if you either want to know as little as possible, or you want to be told everything. But what if you want your communication to fall somewhere in between? Be aware that there's nothing wrong with saying something such as, "Do me a favor. I really want all the information about my case. But please remember that I'm very sensitive, so try to say it to me as gently as possible!"

Explain Your Role in Treatment

At the beginning of a new relationship with a doctor, be sure to clearly explain the kind of role you want to play in your treatment. Some people want to be very active in their treatment. Others want to find somebody they have confidence in, and then let that person run the show. Either approach is fine, depending on your preferences. Make sure not only that you communicate this to your doctor, but also that your doctor, too, is comfortable with the arrangement. This is vital if the relationship is to survive, and if it is to serve you in the best possible way.

GETTING THE MOST FROM OFFICE VISITS

Most of your communications with doctors are likely to take place during office visits. Certainly, you want these visits to be as helpful and productive as possible. But, as you may know, this is sometimes more easily said than done. Probably all of us have at some time come home from a doctor's visit and realized that we forgot to ask an important question. Or perhaps we did ask the question, and then promptly forgot the answer. Nothing can be more frustrating—especially since it is often so difficult to reach a doctor by phone! Fortunately, there are ways in which you can avoid this frustration. Let's look at some of the easy things you can do to get the most from your office visits.

Making a List

Before each appointment, it's important to prepare a list of all the questions you want to ask your doctor. Don't wait until the night before your office visit, though, to put your list together. Instead, prepare the list on an ongoing basis by jotting down notes any time a question or piece of information pops into your mind.

The practice of making a list may seem elementary, but it is an excellent way of obtaining the information you need to understand your condition, properly care for yourself, and guide your treatment. Don't worry that the doctor won't like your preparing a list of questions. Most good doctors do appreciate this practice, because it tends to structure the appointments more efficiently. However, if your doctor doesn't like it, ask yourself this: Whose treatment, condition, and life is on the line?

Besides those questions that occur to you, you may want to include information or questions from family members or close friends, even if you feel that their points may not be important. Your doctor will be able to tell you whether the questions are relevant, as well as provide you with the answers.

Many people worry that the questions they wish to ask are too simple and trivial, or even foolish. Remember that the only foolish question is the unasked question! If you need further explanation of something related to your disorder or treatment, feel free to ask for it, and to be as straightforward in your manner as possible. Ultimately, this will make it easier for your doctor to respond with the information you need.

Getting the Answers

As your doctor answers your questions, be sure to listen carefully. How annoying it is to realize that you've been looking at the next question, rather than listening to the doctor's response! If you're worried that you won't remember everything that goes on in your doctor's office, there are three ways in which you can aid your memory. The first is to jot down notes as the questions are answered. The second is to bring a tape recorder. The third is to bring a family member or close friend.

It can be very helpful to go to the doctor with somebody—not because you need someone to hold your hand, but because two sets of ears are always better than one. Because of the tension most of us feel in the doctor's office, it's easy to miss what's being said. In fact, studies have shown that people remember only a fraction of what their doctor tells them during office visits. Having extra listeners will increase the likelihood that all important information is retained, and will also take some of the pressure off of you, helping you to relax and more efficiently listen and respond. Following the doctor's visit, you and the person who accompanied you will be able to sit down and compare notes about what was said.

If you do decide to bring a family member or friend with you, make sure that this person has a good idea of what you want to accomplish during the appointment. Discuss in advance the kinds of questions you want to ask, and the information you hope to obtain. Your family member will then be able to jump in and ask any questions that he or she feels you've overlooked.

If treatment options are to be discussed during an appointment, consider having several family members attend. In this way, each person in your family will feel that he or she is involved and has input—although, of course, you and your doctor will have the final say as to how you will proceed with your treatment.

Feel free to ask questions about any information your doctor provides during the visit. It is certainly well within your rights to question any aspect of the treatment that is prescribed for you, as well as any medication, any diagnositic procedure, or any other recommendations. Some people, of course, prefer not to ask questions, but to simply follow the dictates of their physician. This, too, is within your rights. But keep in mind that in a situation in which you want to do everything possible to help yourself, the more you know, the better.

Of course, we all want to have confidence in our doctors—to believe that they know what they're talking about. This doesn't mean, however, that you must blindly accept everything your doctor says. For the most part, physicians respect the patient who asks questions. Don't feel that if you disagree, your physician will throw you out. If you are unsure of the reason behind a recommendation, *question it*. It's very important to be honest with your physician—as well as with yourself! If you don't like a particular treatment, or if it does not seem to be working for you, you have the right—in fact, the obligation—to speak up. Being unsure is a certain way to be tense.

It's also important to speak up when you don't understand your doctor's answers because they're too vague or too technical. Don't hesitate to question your doctor further. Perhaps your doctor is used to discussing cases with other doctors, and so has become accustomed to using specialized, scientific terms. Perhaps other patients have been too intimidated to ask for clarifications! Whatever the reason for the problem, don't be afraid to speak up. And don't be embarrassed. Your goal is to talk more comfortably and intelligently about what's happening to you. If you don't understand what's going on or if you don't agree with a treatment plan, let your doctor know.

Other Considerations

What else can you do to make your office visits as profitable as possible? Remember that you're the only one who really knows how you feel. If you think that there is something going on that your doctor should know about, make sure to tell your doctor about it, and make sure that you're heard. Don't think that any piece of information is unimportant, even if the doctor doesn't seem to be as impressed by a particular statement as you expected. Every bit of information that you give can and should help your doctor determine the best course your treatment should take.

Perhaps you're hesitant about giving your doctor all the facts. You might be afraid that you'll be moved to a hospital if your doctor finds out how you're feeling. You might be concerned that your physician won't like the way you've been taking care of yourself. You might fear that your doctor will consider you a complainer who's "crying wolf," and then won't take it seriously when an emergency occurs. Or you might worry that your physician will increase your medication—or *not* increase it! Despite these concerns, you do want your physician to do what's best for you, and this is possible only when you're completely open and honest about the way you've been feeling and how you've been caring for yourself.

While you are at the office, also make sure you have a clear understanding of any medication that has been prescribed for you during the visit. Be certain you know why you should take it, what foods should be eaten—or avoided—along with the medication, and what side effects may be expected. (For more information on medication, see Chapter 18.)

By the time you leave the doctor's office, you will, hopefully, have had your questions answered, and have reached an agreement on your treatment program. By all means, follow this program. This is not to say that if any problems occur as a result of the treatment, they should not be reported. Of course, they should. But, on the other hand, don't expect instantaneous results. Sometimes it can take weeks for your body to respond to a new treatment.

KNOWING WHEN TO CONTACT YOUR DOCTOR

One of the most important questions you'll want to ask your doctor is how you should decide when—and when not—he or she should be called. Which symptoms should be reported immediately? Which symptoms are not as important, and can be reported at the next visit? Ideally, you should get this information as early as possible in your relationship. Ask about the kind of things that should be phoned in, and also ask the best time to call. But when in doubt, check it out. Don't sit by your phone wondering if you should pick it up; just do so. Remember that this is something you've never been through before, so how can you be expected to know exactly what to do? The doctor has been through this many times, so let the doctor tell you that it was not necessary to call at this time (and why!). After you've lived with prostate cancer for a while, you'll have a better idea of when you should call.

While we're discussing when you should contact your doctor, a word should be said about pain. It's vital to clearly communicate to your physician whenever you have pain, and to describe the pain as accurately as possible. Remember that there is no virtue in experiencing pain with cancer. There's no reason for a macho attitude. If you're in pain, tell your doctor, and make sure to get it investigated and, if possible, treated.

GETTING SECOND OPINIONS

Because you may not agree with everything your physician says, and because no physician knows everything, you might want a second opinion. It's always important to get a second opinion if you've been diagnosed with a serious medical problem, or if the prescribed treatment is aggressive—for instance, if surgery has been recommended. This does not necessarily mean that you're questioning the initial diagnosis or prescription for treatment. It simply means that you're wisely exercising caution and seeking to obtain as much information as possible.

Many people worry that if they seek a second opinion, they will hurt their physician's feelings. Are you reluctant to bring up the idea of a second opinion for fear that you'll anger your doctor by appearing to question his or her judgment? Keep your chief priority—your own well-being—in mind, and remember that your doctor is there to treat you and to serve you, but that you're the one who ultimately makes the decisions. In addition, realize that many good physicians will accept— even value—your desire to get a second opinion. In fact, they may take your decision as a matter of course. A good physician will recognize that a second opinion will either confirm what he or she believes, or point out the need for further discussion.

In considering second opinions, here's another fact to keep in mind. Especially after biopsies indicating the presence of cancer, many hospital centers automatically call in additional professionals to offer second opinions regarding both the diagnosis itself and the staging of the cancer. If they feel that this is important, shouldn't you?

Whom Should You Contact?

Certainly, the person you contact for a second opinion should have as much, or more, experience as the first doctor. But how can you locate someone with the proper credentials?

You may start, of course, by asking your family physician or your primary physician for a recommendation. If this doesn't yield the response you're looking for, you can then check with the American Cancer Society, or with the chief of the oncology or urology department in your local hospital. Another resource you might consult is the National Cancer Institute. (See the resource list on page 279.) Or you can check with the medical society of your state or county, which is probably listed in your local telephone book. And, of course, you may wish to seek recommendations from friends—especially from any friends you've made in cancer support groups.

The Second Opinion . . . and Beyond

When you go for a second opinion, make sure to carefully select and prioritize the questions you wish to ask. Keep in mind that it may not be necessary to pose all of the basic questions you asked your initial physician when you were first learning about your disorder. Remember why you're going for the second opinion, and focus on the information that you wish to obtain. Then let the conversation, as well as your written list of questions, guide the way.

If the second opinion significantly differs from the first, you might try to bring the various professionals together to discuss diagnosis and treatment. If this is not possible, however, it may be in your best interest to seek a third opinion. Understandably, you may find this an unappealing option, both because of the pressure it places on you to find another qualified physician and because of financial considerations. Remember, though, that this is your life you're dealing with! So if a third opinion seems to be in order, by all means, get it.

Before we leave the subject of second—and third—opinions, remember that there is a difference between changing physicians and seeking another opinion. A second opinion is sought to validate (or question) your current doctor's diagnosis or prescribed treatment, especially if the disorder is serious or the treatment is extreme. We are not suggesting that you continually shop around for the "ideal" doctor, as no such person exists. We are also not suggesting that you make it a habit to always seek a second opinion. However, when called for, a second opinion can give you the information—and peace of mind—you need to cope with your prostate cancer.

YOU'RE NOT LOCKED IN

Some people have a lot of trouble with the idea of changing physicians. Others seem to change physicians more than they change socks! If you're not happy with your physician, you're not under any obligation to continue seeing him or her. Don't keep going to a particular physician if you feel you can't ask questions, if you feel intimidated, or if you feel that you can't call when there's a problem. Don't stick with your physician if you don't have confidence in the information you're being given, or in the course of treatment that's being prescribed. Finally, don't continue seeing your physician if you feel that he or she doesn't care about you and doesn't have your best interests at heart.

However, before you begin looking for another doctor, carefully examine *why* you want to switch. Are you changing because your doctor does not give you the appropriate information at the appropriate time? Are you changing because the doctor doesn't seem compassionate enough? As far as possible, try to pinpoint the cause of the problem.

After determining what it is that you don't like about your doctor, then attempt to decide if your grievance is *valid*. Be aware that virtually any person who is told that he has prostate cancer will experience anxiety—anxiety that can spill into the doctor-patient relationship, causing problems. Add to this the fact that physicians may not always have the answers—may not always be able to make symptoms or side effects "go away," or to predict the results of a given treatment—and tensions may rise even higher. Is this type of tension affecting your judgment of your doctor? Or is there, in fact, a real problem that must be dealt with?

If the problem is, in fact, valid, you have three options. Option number one is to continue going to your doctor under the present (miserable) conditions. Option number two is to be more assertive, and to discuss the situation with your doctor in the hopes of improving your relationship. Option number three is to simply change doctors without trying to salvage the relationship.

Obviously, number one is not a good option. Staying with a doctor who makes you miserable is not going to contribute to your well-being.

Number two, however, may be worth considering. Many people find that if they talk to their doctor about their concerns in a constructive, positive way, problems can be ironed out. When this is possible, it becomes unnecessary to change doctors. How might you go about approaching your doctor about problems in your relationship? Don't try to accomplish this over the telephone or at the tail end of a regular examination. Instead, set up a separate consultation so that you will have the time to sit down and discuss the things that are worrying you. Once your doctor is made aware of the problem, you may very well be able to reach a mutually satisfactory solution.

Perhaps, though, you don't feel comfortable approaching your doctor in this way. If you are afraid of being honest—or if you feel that your doctor simply can't provide you with the care you need—this relationship may not be the one for you. If so, option number three may be the best choice.

WHEN YOU'RE SEEING SEVERAL DOCTORS

Very likely, during your treatment for prostate cancer, you will be dealing with more than one doctor. As you may have already discovered, this can be a frustrating experience. None of the doctors knows all of the relevant information. Inevitably, there are communication gaps. Even though some of your physicians may work together and try to keep one another informed, there is always something lost in each communication.

Is this a hopeless situation? Absolutely not! When communication gaps exist, you can become the "middleman"—the person who makes sure that each doctor involved has all the necessary information.

First, whenever you are referred to a new doctor, be sure to contact the offices of your present doctors and request that copies of your records be forwarded to the new physician. Then, be sure to keep your own personal anecdotal records, dating back to the time you began dealing with your condition. What should you include in your records? Include all relevant information about your symptoms. List every doctor that you have seen (along with specialty, address, and telephone number), and any diagnoses that have been made by these doctors. Also include a list of all the diagnostic tests that you've received, as well as the results of the tests. Detail all prescribed treatments, describing the results of the treatment, including both the benefits and the side effects. Also record any medications prescribed, including the name, dosage, and side effects, if any. Any other details you feel are important may, of course, also be included.

Keep updating this information, if possible using a word processor so that whenever you see a new doctor, you can easily produce an easy-to-read copy. As time goes by, this information may prove to be invaluable!

IN CONCLUSION

Your goal in life may not have been to be as knowledgeable as possible regarding prostate cancer. Nor is it likely that your goal was to keep ongoing records of your medical history, or to sharpen your communication skills. But you'll find that your efforts in all of these areas will pay big dividends when dealing with doctors—the biggest dividends being greater health and an improved ability to cope with prostate cancer.

Chapter 30

COMMENTS FROM OTHERS

As Ralph Kramden of *The Honeymooners* would say, "Some people have a B-I-G MOUTH!" You may agree with this when you think of some of the comments made by the people around you. They may be close friends or even relatives, but that doesn't mean they know how to talk to you about your condition. They may say things that they think are true, witty, intelligent, or even sympathetic. But you may think otherwise! There may be times when a comment makes you want to implant your knuckles in the speaker's teeth! Or a comment might make you wonder if you're talking to a graduate of the Ignoramus School of Tactlessness.

As you know by now, you cannot change other people. You cannot make them more sensitive or teach them how to be more tactful. But you can learn how to cope with some of the ridiculous comments you hear.

You're probably now eager to learn a few coping strategies. But before we discuss the techniques that will help you cope with annoying comments—and the annoying people who make them—it's important to recognize that most people say things out of sincere concern. They may be trying to make you feel better, to show their support, or to show an interest in you by questioning how you're feeling. Despite the good intentions behind these comments, though, it may not always be possible to respond to them politely and thoughtfully. The problem is that hearing the same questions over and over can get on your nerves. Initially, you may try to gently respond to comments or questions, or to politely change the subject. But this may not always work.

Certainly, some people with prostate cancer avoid unwelcome comments simply by keeping their condition a secret. For the purpose of this chapter, though, let's assume that we're discussing those comments that you can't avoid, made by people who haven't yet learned to tune into your feelings. If you've never experienced any comments of this nature, that's great! But read on anyway. You never know when a tip might come in handy!

HOW SHOULD YOU RESPOND?

Many of the things that people say to you may be legitimate comments, but may bug you just the same. Other remarks may be made without any consideration of your feelings. But it doesn't matter why a comment is inappropriate. What's important is that you handle these comments in a way that makes you feel comfortable.

How might you respond to an annoying comment? There are three ways of responding that might work—that is, that might prevent a further stream of remarks, while making you as comfortable as possible. The first way is to ignore the comment. This is not always easy, especially if the person persistently waits for your answer or seems genuinely insulted by your lack of response. But if you are able to change the subject or walk away, you may get that person to stop asking questions.

The second way of responding to comments is to answer in a rational and intelligent way, explaining how you feel or what you sincerely want to communicate to the other person. This may satisfy the person so that he or she stops making remarks or asking questions. But, of course, there's a limit to the number of times you can explain something, especially if what you're trying to say isn't being understood or accepted. (And this certainly isn't good for your physical health!)

As you see, you may not always be able to cope by ignoring a remark or responding to it rationally. So what can you do when these two approaches fail? You can respond humorously. Why would this work? Well, the person's comment is really unanswerable. So you're going to have a little fun with your response, and humorously let that person know that his or her remark may have been somewhat inappropriate. This technique is called *paradoxical intention*. Let's use the remainder of the chapter to look at some of the comments you may hear, and see how you can use paradoxical intention to answer the unanswerable—without losing your sanity or saying things that you might later regret.

"BUT YOU LOOK SO GOOD!"

It's morning. You've had a full night's sleep, but you're still tired. You have a lot to do to get ready for your day's activities, but you don't feel like doing much of anything. Your wife walks into the room and asks you if you're ready to get up. You tell her that you're not ready yet; you'd like to rest some more because you feel really lousy. She looks at you and says, "How can you feel lousy? You look so good."

Don't you wish you had enough energy to tell her the way you really feel? Any time fatigue drains your muscles of all energy, it can be very frustrating to hear that you should do more because you look so very good. This is one of those statements that's hard to ignore, and just as difficult to answer rationally. So how can you respond to this statement humorously? You might say, "Yes, I know I look good. Remind me to call my plastic surgeon and thank him." Or you can say, "Yes, I look good. It must have been that X-rated dream I had." Notice that in both of these cases, you're first agreeing with the person, and then saying something humorous. Isn't that better than saying, "How can you say I look good when I feel so awful?"

OR "YOU LOOK AWFUL!"

It can be just as upsetting when somebody says, "Wow, you look lousy!" You may feel lousy, but you certainly don't want to be reminded of it. And you surely don't want to think that the way you feel is so obvious to others. You'd like to believe that you at least *look* okay to those around you. Even if it's said sympathetically, this remark may be insulting. So what can you say? You might respond, "Thank you, so do you!" Or, "Yes, I know. I've worked hard to look that way." Or, if you're really in a cynical mood, you might say, "I know I look lousy. That comes from hearing people tell me I look lousy all the time!" Of course, you could always say, "That makes sense, since I don't feel so hot, either!"

"GET BUSY!"

You are quietly sitting in a chair because you feel really exhausted. Somebody comes over to you and asks what's wrong. You try to explain that you're feeling very tired and you're trying to gather some energy. In a concerned way, the person says, "You're spending too much time thinking about yourself. Just get out of that chair and do something. Soon you won't even remember that you're not feeling well!"

How would you react to that? Would you jump out of your chair? Of course not. If you had the energy to get out of your chair, you wouldn't be sitting there in the first place. Would you sit there and try to explain that you're feeling terrible? No, because this person is obviously convinced that you're really feeling fine. You might say, "I would like to get up, but somebody put fast-drying glue on the chair, and I'm stuck forever!" Or you might respond, "I'm trying to set a Guinness World Record for the most time spent sitting in a chair." Or you might say, "Do you know how much energy it takes to remain in this chair, when what I really want to do is get away from you?" Obviously, the type of response you use should depend on how angry or irritated you feel.

Remember: For this approach to work best, you want to keep your tone of voice as light as possible. This will show the person making the comment that you're fine, but that you simply don't appreciate what he or she is saying.

"STOP SEEING SO MANY DOCTORS!"

Let's say that a friend finds out that you have still another doctor's appointment, and remarks, "You're just going to too many doctors. Why don't you stop going all over the place and just take your medication?" How would you respond to this? You might respond by saying, "No. I'd rather keep going to different doctors until I exhaust my bank account." Or you might say, "I like to go to a lot of doctors. The smell of the antiseptic waiting room excites me!" Or, "Do you realize how many of the doctors' children I'm putting through college?"

"WHAT *IS* PROSTATE CANCER?"

How would you respond if somebody sarcastically said, "I never heard of prostate cancer. What is it?" You might say, "Let's forget you even brought it up. Then you can keep your streak going!" Or you could say, "I never heard of it either. How's the weather?" Don't forget: Your aim is not to hurt the other person. However, there are times when being gentle and tactful with others is less important than helping yourself handle comments without becoming aggravated.

What if the person asks why you sound sarcastic? Simply explain that you're not trying to be that way, but that the comment or question you just heard was so ridiculous that you figured the person was trying to be funny. So you decided to have some fun, too! But if the person *really* wants to know how you feel. . . .

"WHAT'S THE MATTER WITH YOUR PROSTATE?"

Some people really don't understand what prostate cancer is all about. (Really!) So they'll bluntly ask you what exactly the problem is with your prostate. This kind of question usually does show genuine concern, so under some circumstances, you might want to simply explain a little more about what prostate cancer is and how it affects you. But if this is the twenty-fourth time you've heard the same question, it may be hard to respond calmly. What could you say that would not be unnecessarily cruel, but would still allow you to feel better about the way you handled the situation—and would, hopefully, end the question-and-answer session? How about, "This isn't my prostate. It's one I borrowed from a neighbor!" Or how about, "Nothing's wrong with my prostate. The local newspaper must have printed an erroneous report!" This is not meant to suggest that you should be unfeeling in your answers. However, if you need to let the "commenter" know that you don't appreciate these questions, this'll do it!

OTHER LOVABLE COMMENTS

What are some of the other comments that you may hear? How many of these have come your way? "Is prostate cancer fatal?" "Why don't you quit your job?" "You should exercise more!" "Are you sure you can walk up those stairs?" "Rest. Don't do anything." "It must hurt to go to the bathroom!" "What is the prognosis?" "Wow, have you changed!" "You must miss the way you used to feel." "I guess you can't have sex, can you?" "Can I help you?" "I certainly don't envy you." "If you ate right, you'd feel better!" "Why don't you try my doctor?" "Your having prostate cancer is the worst thing I ever heard!"

It would fill volumes to include all of the comments that you might hear from "well-meaning" friends or relatives. Hopefully, by reading the previous examples, you've gotten a good idea of how you can respond in a humorous way. Perhaps you'll be able to come up with some additional goodies. Remember that you don't necessarily want to be sarcastic or cruel. Rather, you want to show the speaker that you're feeling well enough to respond with humor and spirit. And you want to show that you can certainly do without this person's helpful bits of information and words of encouragement!

Perhaps you're thinking, "I could never say those things. It's just not my style." Well, you don't always have to. But you can at least *think* these comments. Even that may help you to feel better! And keep in mind that even if you don't want to use this type of response all the time, you may want to use it occasionally, when it seems appropriate to you. And as you learn to more comfortably respond to these comments, you'll find that you can handle these remarks more calmly. Then you'll be able to minimize the sarcasm, and respond with more humorous, enjoyable answers.

A FINAL COMMENT

One of the most common yet upsetting comments has been saved for last. Imagine somebody who is supposedly sympathetic turning to you with eyes full of compassion and concern, saying, "I heard of someone who died from prostate cancer!" As you turn to walk away, you respond, "I heard of someone who died for telling someone with prostate cancer what you just told me!" You walk away, head held high and a smile on your face, leaving the astonished well-wisher behind you.

Chapter 31

SEX AND PROSTATE CANCER

This chapter is not rated *R* for Restricted. Rather, it is rated *E* for Essential. Why? If you are still sexually active, you certainly hope that prostate cancer won't prevent you from having an enjoyable sex life.

There are some people who feel that information about sex is usually not relevant to individuals dealing with prostate cancer, as at advanced ages—the ages during which prostate cancer is most common—the sex drive is virtually nonexistent. Nothing could be further from the truth! Many men at later ages enjoy active sex lives, so concerns about sexual performance are important when coping with prostate cancer.

Has prostate cancer decreased your sexual appetite or ability? Certainly, many people with prostate cancer experience a decreased interest in sex. As a matter of fact, decreased sexual interest is quite common in the presence of a number of chronic medical problems. Is this change likely to be permanent? Well, what kind of sexual relationship did you have before you were diagnosed? (I'm not being nosy. You don't have to write and tell me!) If you had a good sexual relationship, you'll have an easier time getting over any obstacles that prostate cancer may have thrown into your path. If your sexual relationship wasn't good, it is unlikely that having prostate cancer will make it better! You may need some professional help to keep things from breaking down altogether. And if surgery, hormone therapy, or radiation treatments have created problems with performance, alterations may have to be made. But hope is not lost. If you unite with your partner to work things out together, reassure each other, relearn how to please each other, and show a desire for each other, in all likelihood, you can continue to have enjoyable sexual relations.

Sexual problems related to prostate cancer can be physiological or psychological in origin, or can be a combination of the two. Let's look at both types of causes, and at possible means of coping with sexual problems.

PHYSIOLOGICAL PROBLEMS

Can physical problems alter your sexual relations? Yes. Depending on the degree to which prostate cancer or its treatment is affecting you and on your previous level of sexual interest and activity, physical problems may either alter sexual desire or impair sexual performance. Let's learn a little about both of these possibilities.

Decreased Interest

You may think that only psychological factors can affect sexual desire, but various physical problems can also decrease interest in sexual activity. For example, any cancer-related pain or other discomfort—such as nausea or skin irritations—can make it difficult to feel sexual. Fatigue, too, can be a factor. If you're tired, you're going to be less interested in sex. This can be a real headache! (Sorry about that!) Some drugs can also have a direct effect on sexual desire. For example, tranquilizers can suppress sexual desire and also adversely affect your ability to achieve orgasm.

What can you do if your interest in sex has been affected by your prostate cancer? For a time—until your fatigue diminishes, your treatment ends, or other discomforts subside—hanky-panky may just have to be put on hold. Is this a poor choice of words? Actually, it may be an excellent idea. After all, just holding each other can be wonderful, too! If returning to sexual activity following treatment seems uncomfortable or alien, approach things slowly in order to get yourself back into a more normal routine. And be patient. Don't feel that you have to accomplish everything at once. By minimizing the pressure you place on yourself, you can maximize enjoyment and get back into the swing of things at your own pace.

What if your interest in sex fails to increase after a period of time? If a specific drug seems to be the culprit, by all means, speak to your doctor about trying another medication. However, if this doesn't seem to be the solution to your problem, don't hesitate to seek professional guidance.

Impaired Sexual Ability

Certainly, physical problems can impair your sexual function, or even cause impotence. As mentioned earlier, tranquilizers—as well as pain-killers and other drugs—may not only decrease sexual desire, but also reduce the ability to achieve orgasm. Of course, if medication is the problem, your physician may be able to prescribe another drug—one without this side effect. But what about other causes of decreased sexual ability? Let's learn more about impotence, the most extreme form of sexual dysfunction; look at the possible causes of this condition; and explore various ways of dealing with physiological sexual dysfunction.

What Is Impotence?

Impotence, also referred to as sexual or erectile dysfunction, is the inability to achieve and maintain a firm enough erection to permit penetration and intercourse. It is important to note that even when impotence does exist, it may be possible to experience orgasm and to ejaculate, as these activities are controlled by different nerves. In fact, one of the most frustrating aspects of impotence is that desire may continue to be at a high level, even though ability to perform is at a low level.

Interestingly, there are no tests for impotence. Impotence is usually a self-reported symptom. But because of the stigma associated with impotence, many men are reluctant to talk about it, and therefore often deny themselves available help.

What Can Cause Impotence?

As discussed earlier in the book, in the past, radical prostatectomy almost always caused impotence—not as a result of prostate gland removal, but as a result of nerve damage. Today, because of improved surgical techniques—specifically, the retropubic approach—there is less chance of damaging the erection mechanism. (For information on the retropubic approach, see page 37.) However, surgery still sometimes causes nerve damage and a resulting impairment of sexual function.

Radiation therapy, too, may sometimes lead to impotence, as the radiation process itself may result in trauma, scarring, or other types of nerve damage. And hormone therapy—whether through orchiectomy or hormone suppression—can lead to both a decrease in sexual desire and impotence.

Of course, intercourse is not the only means of deriving sexual pleasure. One of the goals of individuals who have experienced irreversible physical damage is the exploration and enjoyment of other means of sexual expression. But if you have lost and now seek to regain full sexual function, read on!

Improving Sexual Performance

There are a number of devices and medications that can help you cope with impotence. These aids permit erection, penetration, and intercourse.

Penile Implants. Since the 1970s, surgeons have been able to implant objects in the penis to enable an effective erection. These devices fall into one of two categories. The first includes semi-rigid prostheses, and the second includes inflatable and hydraulic devices.

The first modern semi-rigid device used—and one that is still used, although rarely—is the Small-Carrion penile prosthesis. This device, made of silicone tubes containing spongy material, is inserted in the penis, causing a permanent semi-rigid erection. Intercourse, is, of course, facilitated by this implant. However, many men do not like this device simply because the erection is permanent.

Another semi-rigid device is the Flexi-Rod implant. This is similar to the Small-Carrion prosthesis, but has hinged rods instead of solid ones, allowing the penis to hang more naturally for better concealment. Intercourse is possible with this implant as well, but some men have reported a little more difficulty in achieving penetration. This device, like the Small-Carrion, is now seldom used because of the advent of the inflatable prostheses.

Inflatable prostheses are made up of a number of components—hollow cylinders, a pump, a reservoir, and connecting tubes. The cylinders are implanted in the penis, while the fluid-filled reservoir is located under the scrotum, beneath the skin. When the man wants to achieve an erection, he presses the pump. This fills the cylinders with fluid, in much the way the penis normally fills with blood during sexual activity. After orgasm, the pump valve is released, returning the fluid to the reservoir, and the penis to its normally flaccid state. Hydraulic prostheses work in much the same way, and both types of devices allow the genitals to retain a natural appearance.

You may be frightened by the prospect of surgical implantation. As with any surgery, there will be discomfort, and a period of recovery will be necessary. The possibility of infection also exists, although it is not a common occurrence. How long will you have to wait before you can use your new equipment? It is usually estimated that you can begin enjoying sex approximately four to six weeks after surgery.

Perhaps even more important than recovery time is the final result. Do these prostheses provide the same pleasure during sex as would be experienced with normal physical function? The news here is good. In most cases, the implants enable the user to enjoy normal sexual relations.

If you are considering penile implants, you should think carefully about a number of factors. For instance, how do you feel about having a foreign object in your body? Is cost a factor? (The inflatable prostheses tend to cost more than the semi-rigid devices.) If you're married or have a regular sexual partner, your partner should also be involved in the decision-making process. Sometimes, a man decides on his own to have an implant, only to find after surgery that the woman in his life is so turned off by the device that she is no longer interested in sex. It is essential that all decisions focus on desirability—not simply availability.

Nonsurgical Devices. There are a number of nonsurgical alternatives to implants, including, most notably, external vacuum devices. These devices contain a cylinder that is placed over the penis. A pump connected by tube to the cylinder draws air from the cylinder either by mouth or automatically, creating a vacuum around the penis. This results in increased blood flow to the penis, causing an erection. The vacuum is then released, the cylinder is removed, a special rubber band is placed at the base of the penis to maintain the erection, and intercourse can begin. An electric pump, which has a similar effect, is also available.

A major disadvantage to the use of both of these devices is that they are visible to both partners, which can be a turn-off. As a result, the pumps are less widely used than are injections.

Injections. Currently, the most commonly used method of inducing an erection is the injection of certain drugs into the penis. Although the very idea of this may make some people cringe, this method is highly effective, and, in fact, causes little or no pain.

Papaverine and Regitine (phentolamine mesylate), which have been used to treat heart disease for many years, both have the effect of causing an erection when injected into the side of the penis. After intercourse, the erection quickly fades. The effectiveness of these self-administered injections has caused a significant decrease in the number of men who undergo surgery for the implantation of prostheses.

At this time, a combination of papaverine, Regitine, and the prostaglandins—homonelike fatty acids—is being used with great success. This "cocktail" seems to decrease the side effects of the individual drugs—used alone, some of the drugs cause scarring or burning—while maximizing results.

Researchers are now working to develop external preparations of papaverine and Regitine—preparations that can be rubbed on the skin. A urethral suppository is also being investigated. By the time you read this book, new, more convenient products may be available.

PSYCHOLOGICAL PROBLEMS

What's your most important sexual organ? Think hard now. The correct response is—your brain! So if a sexual problem has no physiological cause, then its cause is psychological. In fact, the psychological variables that affect sexual activity are just as real as the physiological factors. Anxiety, depression, and fear can all form emotional blocks that severely impair sexual performance.

Let's learn about various psychological problems that may affect sexual relations, and discuss how these obstacles can be overcome.

Poor Self-Image

Living with prostate cancer can certainly affect your self-esteem. Do you feel like a different person now that you have prostate cancer? Do you feel as if you're no longer physically intact? If your answer to either of these questions is "Yes," you may be more fearful of rejection by your partner. As a result, you may reduce sexual activity simply to minimize the chance of rejection.

There are many reasons why you may perceive yourself as being different as a result of your cancer. For instance, if you've had surgery, you may feel a real sense of loss. You may not be able to see what you lost—and nobody else may be able to see it, either. Nevertheless you may feel less attractive or less sexual, and more self-conscious.

Other Emotional Interference

Sexual activity—and sexual desire—may be impaired by a number of emotions. For instance, depression may keep you from having any interest in sex. Anxiety concerning the sex itself or your condition may also decrease desire or affect performance. You may be afraid that you just can't "make it." Or you may be afraid that sexual activity will exacerbate any prostate cancer symptoms you're experiencing. You might even fear that sexual relations will create new symptoms. (There is no basis for this fear!)

Among the psychological concerns that may lead to erectile problems is the fact that many older men are not aware that advancing age results in an increase in the amount of time necessary both to become aroused and to ejaculate. As a result, they may feel that the need for more time is a result not of age, but of the cancer or the cancer's treatment. Because they think that a problem exists, they become fearful, and fear of poor performance leads to poor performance.

What You Can Do

When psychological problems affect sexual desire or performance, it's necessary to get at the root of the problem, and to use coping strategies to eliminate the troubling emotions. For instance, let's say that you've realized that prostate cancer has made you feel like less of a person sexually—a common reaction—and that this is the cause of your sexual worries. You've now targeted an important area on which to work. Try to remember that nobody's perfect. Everybody has flaws. Then work on increasing your feelings of self-esteem.

If anxiety or depression is affecting your sexual well-being, you'll want to improve your attitude and combat the troubling emotion. Use some of the thought-changing procedures described earlier in the book. They may be the key to your future happiness!

What else can you do to eliminate psychological obstacles to a fulfilling sex life? A very important part of sexual relationships is communication. If you and your partner can share thoughts and feelings, you'll be in much better shape to work out any problems that may occur as a result of your condition.

What might you talk about with your partner? Acknowledge and discuss any sexual fears or problems. If necessary, work to alter the ways in which the two of you express your sexual desires. Fully communicate your needs and desires. For instance, if there are times when you're just too tired for sexual activity, feel free to tell your partner about your fatigue. And remember that problems get worse only when you chronically avoid the issues—not when you openly discuss them and work together to find solutions.

Besides communicating your feelings and fears to your partner, you might also want to discuss any problems with your physician or with other health professionals. For instance, if you're concerned that sexual activity will worsen your symptoms, your doctor will probably be able to allay your fears.

Everything that's been said in this section assumes that your sexual interest or performance has been affected by psychological problems, and that your partner is suffering as a result. But what if the opposite is true? What if you still have normal sexual desires and normal performance, but your partner is the one who's afraid? Perhaps she's fearful of creating additional problems. Perhaps she regards you as being fragile simply because you have cancer, and is reluctant to initiate or respond to sexual overtures. Discuss this with your partner. Make sure that you communicate with each other, and be sure to set up ground rules so that you know which sexual activities are okay and which (if any) aren't. And if these one-on-one attempts at working things out don't help, don't hesitate to get some professional assistance. The results will be well worth the effort.

IN CONCLUSION

When dealing with any sexual problems that result from your prostate cancer, remember that much can be done to improve your sexual functioning as well as your feelings regarding sex. As a matter of fact, in many cases, sex can be as pleasurable and important as both partners want it to be. Physical and medical aids and psychological coping strategies can help you overcome most obstacles to interest and performance. But most important is open communication with your partner. Even if your sex life becomes less active, you can still have a warm relationship—but not if there are bitter feelings and misgivings. Honest discussions, marked by understanding, are a vital part of coping with sexual problems, just as they are a necessary part of coping with all aspects of prostate cancer.

Chapter 32

LIVING WITH SOMEONE WITH PROSTATE CANCER

Any medical problem as serious as prostate cancer doesn't affect just the person with the disease. It also affects everyone who's close to that person—family members and friends. Those who are in the inner circle, and especially those who live with the patient, are affected in the most significant way. They are also in the best position to help the person who is living with prostate cancer.

Illness can create troubling changes in relationships. (No kidding!) If you live with someone who has prostate cancer, you may now see that person—and even yourself—differently. Maybe you see that person as being more fragile. Maybe their disorder has reminded you of your own vulnerability. Maybe you somehow feel guilty about their condition, or about your feelings regarding the condition. Maybe you were formerly quite dependent on that person, and you now have to shoulder more responsibility.

What does all this mean? First, you have concerns regarding the individual who has prostate cancer. And you feel responsible for his welfare. Certainly, more and more research has shown that when a person has cancer, his will to live, his outlook, his self-confidence, his acceptance of his condition, and his desire for recovery are important factors in outcome. You want to do everything you can to enhance all of these factors—and to provide that person with all necessary practical assistance as well. But there may be times when it's very difficult for you to provide this help. There may be times when you must reach out and get your own help so that you can be as strong as you possibly can for that person.

This chapter will first look at what you can do to help your loved one. It will then look at what you can do to help yourself cope with the problems involved in caring for a person with prostate cancer. (By the way, thoughout this book, I have purposely avoided calling the person with prostate cancer a "patient," simply because I believe in emphasizing the person rather than the condition. However, for the sake of convenience and because repeating "your loved one" can become tedious, in this chapter, I will sometimes refer to the person with prostate cancer as the patient.)

HOW YOU CAN HELP THE PATIENT WITH PROSTATE CANCER

If you are close to someone with prostate cancer, you have an important job on your hands—a job made up of many components. But what exactly is your job, and how can you best fill it? Read on!

Maintain Normalcy

When spending time with your loved one, try to behave much as you've always behaved with this person. Try to minimize any changes in your interactions. This isn't meant to suggest that you should not acknowledge, through word or deed, that the person has cancer. As we will discuss later in the chapter, it's vital to be open about feelings, and to honestly discuss any problems. Just try not to dwell on the patient's condition.

Why is it so important to maintain normalcy? Well, finding out that you have cancer can be shocking enough, and worries about the way in which the condition will change everyday life are also upsetting. By keeping life as normal as possible, you'll help to compensate for the many changes that must take place and give the person a stronger sense of security.

Prevent Isolation

People with prostate cancer usually have to face many problems, both physical and emotional in nature. These problems are even harder to deal with when patients feel alone and isolated. Yet, in some cases, even a person who has many friends can become isolated as a result of prostate cancer. Why? A lot of people are so uncomfortable being around someone with cancer that they find every excuse possible to avoid contact, rationalizing this behavior by telling themselves that there are so many other people around that they don't have to visit or call. Still others don't intentionally avoid the person with cancer, but make no special effort to see him when restrictions keep him from participating in his usual activities.

Fortunately, as a person who's close to the patient, you may be able to help. Do what you can to preserve the connection between your loved one and his friends and relatives. Speak to those people who seem to have dropped out of sight. See if there is anything you can do to reestablish these important relationships.

In some cases, of course, rather than fading away, relationships may become stronger than ever. Friends and family members may provide much-needed emotional support, and also offer rides to the hospital, cooked meals, and other practical help. This is a wonderful blessing. But be careful not to take advantage of others' generosity. Make sure that nothing happens to burn out these invaluable relationships.

Become a Loyal Learner

You can help the patient a great deal simply by learning as much as you can about prostate cancer and its treatment. The knowledge you obtain will allow you to provide support and true understanding—both of which are boons to the person with prostate cancer. Knowing the facts may help you, as well, as it may dissipate any fear of the unknown, and help eliminate your confusion over symptoms, treatments, and side effects.

Encourage, Don't Pester

Certainly, you should encourage your loved one to adhere to proper treatment routines. But don't badger. If the patient is not taking proper care of himself, there is a limit to what you can do to change his behavior. Screaming usually doesn't help. (And it can hurt your vocal cords!)

If the patient is not taking care of himself, should you tell his physician? That's a hard question to answer. You don't want to overstep your bounds, as this may lead to resentment on the part of the patient. At the same time, especially if your loved one doesn't seem to care about his welfare, you don't want to sit back and let him create unnecessary problems.

So what should you do? Play it by ear. Voice your concerns to the patient, explaining that you're afraid of any problems becoming worse due to lack of treatment. Then carefully listen to his response before deciding whether to contact his physician or take other steps.

Provide Support, Not Pity

Because of the difficulties of living with prostate cancer and its treatment, you may sympathize with the patient. You may feel sad about what he has to go through. The sympathy you feel may help you provide beneficial support. But don't pity the patient, as this can be destructive.

Be aware that treatment for prostate cancer—whether surgery, radiation, or hormone therapy—can affect mood, causing depression. Try to prepare yourself for these bouts of depression, and try to resist any temptation to run away from the patient. Prostate cancer is not contagious, and your loving support may be one of the most important factors in the patient's emotional state. How, exactly, can you help? If you sense that your loved one is wallowing in self-pity, you may be able to help him by joining him—not necessarily by crying, but by just being there, reaching out, and touching him. Sometimes, just by listening and allowing the patient to express his feelings, you can turn negative emotions into positive ones. Don't feel that you have to quickly snap him out of his depression. A certain amount of self-pity can be a constructive self-indulgence. Problems exist only when the period of self-pity continues too long. If this happens, do what you can to restore the patient's spirits, consulting a professional if necessary.

During times of depression, you will probably want to be as encouraging as possible. But avoid giving the patient false hope or false promises. It's not always wonderfully reassuring to hear that "everything will be fine." On occasion, this comment can cause more harm than good by making the patient lose faith in your honesty and candor.

There will be times when the patient is so fatigued that he can do little or nothing. At such times, it is not appropriate for you to insist that he "get up and do something." That won't make him feel better. Instead, try to help him out by taking over some of his obligations and responsibilities. This may help reduce any pressure he feels, and will certainly allow him to better conserve energy. But, at the same time, don't allow the patient to baby himself. In general, if he can do something—even if it takes some time for him to do it—let him. If you feel that the patient is malingering, by all means, discuss it with him. Try to make life as normal as possible for him.

As the cancer progresses, your loved one may become more passive and lethargic. He may seem to gradually lose hope, and therefore be less willing to participate in normal activities. You can help him by encouraging him to remain involved in normal activities, and to do as much as he is physically able to do.

Avoid Overprotection

As a family member or close friend, it's very important to tune into the needs of your loved one. Do not assume that you should be overprotective or underprotective simply because that's the way you would want others to act if you were ill. Be sure to find out what the patient wants, and try as much as possible to act accordingly.

For example, you may feel that you want to protect your loved one by keeping him in the dark regarding the severity of the disease or the possible side effects of a treatment option. Protect him from this information only if he has clearly communicated to you that this is what he wants. You may want to discuss this with him as soon as possible, and to ask him every now and then if he has changed his mind about what he wants to be told.

Don't stay on top of the patient. Sure, you want to help. When he's tired, for instance, you want to relieve him of some of his chores. But give him sufficient space to regain some control over his own life. How? When he's no longer tired, be sure to let him resume his normal activities. Don't tell him to get into bed and rest! Have faith in your special someone. If he really doesn't feel well, he will rest. Otherwise, let him be.

Many people become especially overprotective—and sometimes downright pushy!—when food is concerned. Don't feel that you should push the patient to eat when he doesn't want to. Yes, it's important for a person with cancer to eat a nutritionally sound diet, but if you push too hard, you may simply make him more resistant to your suggestions. And, anyway, you don't want to be seen as a nag!

What about accompanying the patient on doctors' visits? If your loved one agrees, you may want to go along for the ride. It's an excellent idea to have four ears, rather than two, listening when the doctor explains the prostate cancer itself or details treatment options. However, if the patient wants to go alone, and feels strongly about it, don't force him to take you with him.

What's the bottom line here? As soon as possible, work with your loved one to set ground rules. Hopefully, he will initiate this. If not, you can start the discussion. Talk about your interest in being as supportive as you possibly can, and ask what you can do to help. Things will move more smoothly once you have a good idea of what to do and when to do it. Even if no clear-cut answers emerge, at least you'll share some constructive communication, which will lay the groundwork for handling future problems. Perhaps most important—and, possibly, most difficult—try to respect the patient's decisions regarding how he wants things handled. Discussions are fine, but ultimately, he has to make the final decisions.

Keep Talking!

What's the best way to talk to your loved one? Unfortunately, because everybody's different—and because needs change along with moods and circumstances—there's no way to know for sure. At certain times, you may feel that it's best to respond with sympathy and understanding. At other times, it may be best to just ignore the situation and walk away. To a degree, you'll have to play things by ear, remaining as attuned to the patient as possible.

However you decide to talk to the patient, by all means, *keep talking*. The most important key to the successful maintenance of family harmony is communication. Perhaps good communication patterns were in place in your family prior to the diagnosis of prostate cancer. If so, you're one of the lucky ones. If not, it's imperative to open the lines of communication and keep them open.

Why is good communication so important? Only through communication will you learn how the patient feels, both physically and emotionally. And only by knowing how he feels will you be able to help him. This doesn't mean that the conversations will always be pleasant. Talking about treatment problems, depression, fears, or pain isn't very enjoyable, especially if you don't have solutions to the problems. But with good communication, any difficulties will be overshadowed by the feeling of closeness that results from shared experiences and concerns.

As much as you would like to talk to your loved one, there may be times when he is not willing to respond. When this happens, it's perfectly okay to reassure him that you're aware that he doesn't want to talk right now, but that you'll be there for him when he needs a sympathetic ear.

At times, you may feel that it would be helpful to ask your loved one how *you* can cope with the difficulty of the situation—with the uncertainties you feel about how you can help him, and with your own fears about his condition. Certainly, there's nothing wrong with pointing out that you're concerned. Make sure you do it at an appropriate time, though. And if you see that the subject is upsetting the patient, put the conversation on hold.

TAKE CARE OF YOURSELF, TOO!

Although you probably learned a great deal about the experience of prostate cancer from reading earlier chapters of this book, we have so far paid little attention to the problems prostate cancer poses for those who care for the patient. There are many times when a family member has a harder time dealing with illness than does the person who is ill. You may experience many of the same emotions and changes in lifestyle experienced by the patient, but feel more helpless and out of control because everything is happening *around* you rather than *to* you. In addition, there are special problems that you will encounter as one who is probably responsible for much of the patient's care. Let's take a look at some of the problems you may face, and see how you can care not only for the patient, but also for an equally important person—yourself!

Guilt

In Chapter 14, we discussed how your loved one may experience guilt as a result of his prostate cancer. But you, too, may be troubled by this emotion. You may feel (irrationally) that you somehow contributed to the patient's cancer. You may feel that you should have been more insistent about his seeing a doctor when problems first occurred. You may feel guilty because, although you're concerned about the patient, you resent the fact that his illness is going to interfere with the quality of your life. This last thought may make you feel especially bad, as your anger and resentment are directed towards somebody who, at the present time, is vulnerable and unable to defend himself.

How can you cope with your feelings of guilt? Work to restructure your own thinking, just as the patient who experiences guilt must restructure his. Keep reminding yourself that you did not cause the cancer. You are not a bad person. You are are doing what you can to help your loved one. By reworking your negative thoughts, you will be able to reduce any feelings of guilt that might arise.

Depression

Just as the patient will sometimes feel depressed, you should anticipate that you, too, will sometimes experience depression. Accept that it's okay to feel this way. After all, it's certainly depressing when treatment doesn't seem to bring about the desired results. However, this depression should not be allowed to linger. Techniques should be used to lift the depression to at least some degree.

Again, begin by restructuring your thinking. Depression is often caused by negative thoughts, so you'll want to follow the suggestions provided in Chapter 11 for changing those thoughts. In addition, make sure to leave some time in each day for yourself. It is essential to have time in which you can do the things you enjoy. This isn't being selfish or negligent. Rather, by helping yourself, you'll be making yourself stronger and better able to support your loved one.

The Long Versus the Short of It

When someone experiences an acute (short-term) medical problem—
such as major surgery or a broken bone—it's relatively easy for friends
and relatives to rally around, provide support and understanding, and
temporarily take over responsibilities. But a condition such as prostate
cancer is a different matter. There will be times when your loved one
may be able to do very little, and you will have to take on many more
chores. At other times, the patient will be able to do a lot more, and you
and other family members will have to readjust and allow him to resume
more of his former routine. These cyclical changes can create major
problems. And the fact that there is no definite time when the problem
will end will not make your adjustment any easier.

How can you cope with problems caused by the long-term nature of
prostate cancer? Once again, work on your thinking. Long-range worries
lead to long-term unhappiness. Instead of thinking about the future, do
what you can each day to help your loved one and to make his life and
your own as full and happy as possible. Have faith in your ability to rise
to new challenges if and when it becomes necessary to do so.

A Final Note on Self-Care

You know that the person with prostate cancer needs care and support.
But don't ignore the fact that you, too, need—and deserve—nurturing
and caring attention. Don't be afraid to reach out and get it. Don't feel
that because you're not the person who is sick, you have to take a back
seat. Your emotions can suffer as well. Remember that you can benefit
from the same kinds of support groups that can help your loved one.
Don't hesitate to take advantage of them. For you to continue to be at
your best for yourself, for your loved one, and for other members of your
family, you need to be strong.

A SUPPORTIVE CONCLUSION

True, prostate cancer is not affecting your body. But it certainly is
affecting you in other ways. By following the suggestions in this chapter,
you can help yourself be stronger, more emotionally stable, and more
supportive of your loved one. After all, he's not the only one who has to
cope with prostate cancer!

ON TO THE FUTURE

Well, you've just about finished this book. We've covered a lot of information about prostate cancer. Ongoing research continues to test new medical techniques that may be able to treat the condition, as well as further improve the quality of life for people with prostate cancer.

Perhaps by the time you read this, some drug or treatment may have proven itself to be even more successful than the ones discussed within these pages. It remains to be seen which new developments may improve your life with prostate cancer. But it's nice to know that people continue to work on the problem.

Although it would be impossible to discuss every conceivable problem related to prostate cancer, I hope that what you've read will help you develop your own strategies for coping. Because things change, and something that troubles you one day may not trouble you the next (and vice versa), this book should be used as a resource. Whenever you have questions about how to cope with a certain aspect of prostate cancer, consult these pages. If you have any comments, information you feel is important, or additional questions, feel free to write to me in care of Avery Publishing Group, 120 Old Broadway, Garden City Park, New York 11040.

Until such time as there no longer is a medical condition called prostate cancer, keep coping the best you can. Remember that despite prostate cancer, you can *always* improve the quality of your life.

But for now, look brightly ahead, act proudly, and enjoy life as best you can. I wish all of my readers the very best of health and happiness!

FOR FURTHER READING

The following books—which provide more information on the material presented in this book, and focus on other topics, as well—may help you cope with various aspects of living with prostate cancer. By no means should you limit yourself to the books listed below. Many other publications also examine cancer treatment, nutrition, the challenges of living with chronic illness, and other subjects that may be of interest to you. Don't hesitate to take advantage of all the information available to you at your local library and bookstore.

Betler, R., and Lewis, M. *Love and Sex After Forty.* New York: Harper and Row Publishers, 1986.

Dollinger, M. et al. *Everyone's Guide to Cancer Therapy: How Cancer Is Diagnosed, Treated, and Managed on a Day to Day Basis.* Kansas City, MO: Andrews and McMeel, 1991.

Fanning, P. *Visualization for Change.* Oakland, CA: New Harbinger Publications, 1988.

Fink, J. *Third Opinion: An International Directory to Alternative Therapy Centers for the Treatment and Prevention of Cancer and Other Degenerative Diseases.* Garden City Park, NY: Avery Publishing Group, 1992.

Fiore, N. *The Road Back to Health: Coping With the Emotional Side of Cancer.* New York: Bantam Books, 1984.

Greenberger, M., and Siegel, M. *What Every Man Should Know About His Prostate.* New York: Walker Publishing, 1983.

Holleb, A. *The American Cancer Society Cancer Book: Prevention, Detection, Diagnosis, Treatment.* New York: Doubleday, 1986.

Jochems, R. *Dr. Moermon's Anti-Cancer Diet: Holland's Revolutionary Pro-*

gram for Combating Cancer. Garden City Park, NY: Avery Publishing Group, 1990.

Kubler-Ross, E. *On Death and Dying.* New York: Macmillan, 1970.

Kushi, A., and Esko, W. *The Macrobiotic Cancer Prevention Cookbook.* Garden City Park, NY: Avery Publishing Group, 1988.

Kushi, M., with Esko, E. *The Macrobiotic Approach to Cancer: Towards Preventing and Controlling Cancer With Diet and Lifestyle.* Garden City Park, NY: Avery Publishing Group, 1991.

Lane, I., and Comac, L. *Sharks Don't Get Cancer: How Shark Cartilage Could Save Your Life.* Garden City Park, NY: Avery Publishing Group, 1993.

Lazarus, A. *In the Mind's Eye.* New York: Rawson Associates, 1977.

Matthews-Simonton, S., and Shook, R. *The Healing Family.* Bantam Books, 1984.

Simone, C. *Cancer and Nutrition: A Ten-Point Plan to Reduce Your Risk of Getting Cancer.* Garden City Park, NY: Avery Publishing Group, 1992.

Simonton, O., Matthews-Simonton, S., and Creighton, J. *Getting Well Again.* Bantam Books, 1978.

Walters, R. *Options: The Alternative Cancer Therapy Book.* Garden City Park, NY: Avery Publishing Group, 1993.

RESOURCE GROUPS

The following groups can provide you with more information on prostate cancer, suggest helpful books and videos, direct you to support groups, and inform you of other valuable services. Feel free to contact these organizations and benefit from their expertise.

American Cancer Society (ACS)
1599 Clifton Road, N.E.
Atlanta, GA 30329
(800) ACS–2345
(404) 320–3333

Canadian Cancer Society
130 Bloor Street West
Suite 1001
Toronto, Ontario,
Canada M5S 2V7
(416) 961–7223

Cancer Care, Inc.
1180 Avenue of the Americas
New York, NY 10036
(212) 719–9421

National Cancer Institute
Cancer Information Service (CIS)
National Institutes of Health
Building 31, Room 10A24
Bethesda, MD 20892
(800) 422–6237

INDEX